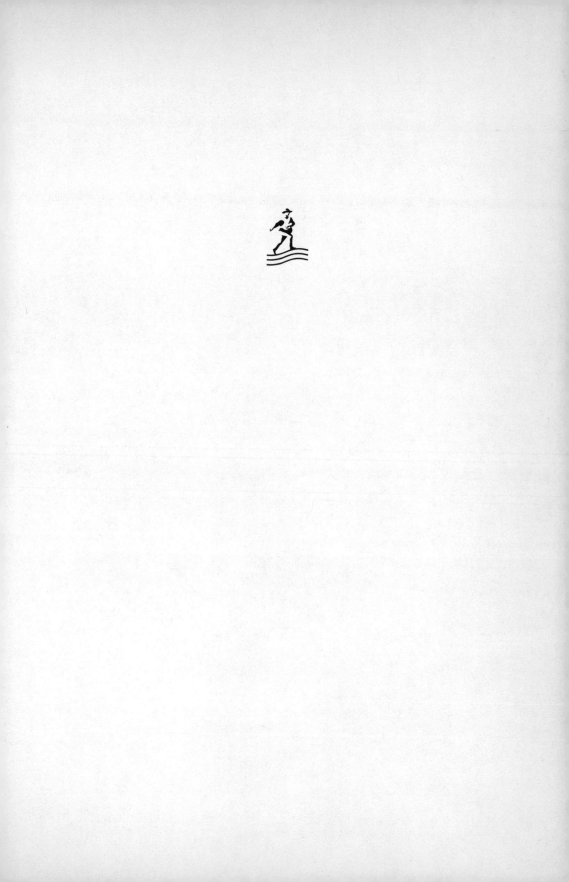

ALSO BY NAOMI JUDD

*Naomi's Breakthrough Guide:*
*Twenty Choices to Transform Your Life*

*Love Can Build a Bridge* (autobiography)

*Naomi's Home Companion*

# NAOMI JUDD

# NAOMI'S
## GUIDE TO AGING
# GRATEFULLY

*Facts, Myths, and Good News*
*for Boomers*

SIMON & SCHUSTER
New York   London   Toronto   Sydney

SIMON & SCHUSTER
Rockefeller Center
1230 Avenue of the Americas
New York, NY 10020

For information regarding special discounts for bulk purchases,
please contact Simon & Schuster Special Sales at 1-800-456-6798
or business@simonandschuster.com.

*Designed by Joel Avirom and Jason Snyder*

Manufactured in the United States of America

10   9   8   7   6   5   4   3   2   1

Library of Congress Cataloging-in-Publication Data

Judd, Naomi.
    [Guide to aging gratefully]
    Naomi's guide to aging gratefully : facts, myths, and good news for boomers /
Naomi Judd.
        p.   cm.
    Includes bibliographical references.
    1. Older people—Psychology.    2. Older people—Conduct of life.
3. Middle-aged persons—Psychology.    4. Middle-aged persons—Conduct
of life.    5. Baby boom generation.    6. Aging—Psychological aspects.
7. Self-actualization (Psychology)   8. Self-perception.    I. Title.
II. Title: Guide to aging gratefully.
HQ1061.J83   2007
646.7008'4—dc22                                                      2006052217

ISBN-13: 978-0-7432-7515-6
ISBN-10:    0-7432-7515-2

*Have you been feeling anxiety about your maturing appearance
and changing body shape and dreading birthdays?
Do you find yourself lamenting the way you looked ten years ago
and constantly comparing yourself to women in the media?
This book is written for you. Perception is everything,
and yours is about to improve.*

# CONTENTS

# NAOMI'S
## GUIDE TO AGING
# GRATEFULLY

"If every day is an awakening, you will never grow old. You will just keep growing."

—GAIL SHEEHY, AUTHOR OF *PASSAGES*

# 1 | *All About Eve:* The Birth of a Notion

I GOT THE DETERMINATION to write *Aging Gratefully* after *Grand* magazine named me one of the top ten sexiest grandparents in the world. The list included Mick Jagger, Pierce Brosnan, Goldie Hawn, and Harrison Ford. I was proud to be included in what was a celebration of aging, and proof positive that Baby Boomers can be vital, exciting, healthy, productive, and yes, even *sexy* in their later years 'cause that's how I feel.

But the notion had already been brewing from my disquiet at society's growing prejudice against aging. Every time we see someone over fifty (if we see them at all) on television or in magazines, they're typically marginalized, or somehow portrayed as feeble or useless. Nothing could be farther from the truth! The first time Wy and I went to the fun house at the state fair while performing as the Judds, we were bemused at our grotesque images in the fun-house mirrors. But now this is how society's distorted reflection of aging feels today. Wy and I kept bumping into mirrors trying to navigate the maze. Suddenly we almost collided and Wy raised her hand to my face. Wondering aloud, she asked, "Are you real?"

## Being Real

The number one cause of mental illness and unhappiness is not knowing who you are. This book is about looking in the mirror of truth and realizing and embracing who you are in mind and body and spirit. So instead of the most expensive over-the-counter cream or a visit to a plastic surgeon, think of these choices as your most effective weapon against *fear* of aging. Grab your bifocals or magnifying glasses and let's learn our options. I'm going to show you Grandma ain't what she used to be.

My friend Lily Tomlin says, "Anyone who writes a self-help book should first be able to prove they've helped themselves." So to begin every chapter, I'll reveal the personal story of my own experiences through the years. First I want to introduce you to a girl from my past named Naomi (name not a coincidence, as you will soon discover). She was a fellow student at Crabbe Grade School in Ashland, Kentucky. She was slow and unlovely. Every day I watched as Naomi walked by herself to our old stone schoolhouse. By contrast, as long as I can remember, people have told me how pretty I am. Seems it's only served to make me even more aware of how little external appearances mean. I didn't do anything to earn the looks or IQ with which I was born. Neither did Naomi. Neither did you.

We didn't get to choose the body or face with which we are born. Nor can we stop time from moving on. Somehow, even when I was in my early twenties, I intuited that basic reality. Maybe it was because I was in Hollywood, where I was becoming more and more upset about seeing people, especially women, allow themselves to be defined by our ever-changing, superficial culture. Thank goodness I began looking inward for my identity. I immediately felt less desperate. I realized that whenever I look at the fun-house mirror of society, I can remember it's only a distortion.

As I searched to figure out my values, I realized I value helping others. I left Hollywood to move us to Kentucky. My inner knowing steered me toward choosing to go to college and get a nursing degree. I valued a career in which character and caring matter more than the gift of genes. My patients didn't care what my face looked like, how old I was, or how much I weighed.

Shift happens. With this shift in my awareness, I felt more confident and more and more in control of my true self-image. I felt so much better about my future! I even went so far as to change my name from Diana Ellen Judd to Naomi Ellen Judd. Looking back, this early decision to change my first name, in recognition of that other Naomi (who still reminds me to be grateful) has helped preserve my sanity. I couldn't predict in the seventies that I would later be getting into the grandmother of all superficial and vain careers, showbiz. Somehow I have found my way in this most ageist of professions. I'm happier today at sixty-one than I've ever been. The critical steps I've learned along my journey are the ones I'm eager to share with you, dear reader.

It was a life-affirming breakthrough when I saw I could choose not to allow the culture, media, and some ad agency to impose harmful, unrealistic views and ideas about beauty, size, and age on me. Ever since then, I'm okay with growing older. I see it as something I'm going toward, rather than something to run away from. You can't stop the river, let's go with the flow. I've had a lot of ups and downs in my life—married and with a child at eighteen, struggles with money and inappropriate men as a single mom, fame, fortune, and marriage to a wonderful man in my late thirties, forced retirement due to a supposed terminal illness in my late forties, and then the reinvention of myself as an author and a speaker, and with my own TV show in my fifties. I've survived so much stuff that my personal history (her story) is a testament to how not to sweat the stuff that's out of your control. When I can't control outer circumstances, I choose to change your reaction. That means you and I can change our reaction to aging too.

Aging is one of those things that you just can't control. As you and I grow older, changes in our physical appearance, as well as our mental capacity, are inevitable. Entropy isn't what it used to be (pun intended). We can't bargain with the clock, but we can react by making the best choices. One most important choice is to choose to be at peace with ourselves *exactly* as we are.

In this uncertain time of post 9/11, we certainly have enough to be insecure about. You and I don't need to be worrying about sagging bust lines and crow's-feet. I want to show you, whatever your age, that you can feel great, live fully, and be comfortable with and even embrace aging. So many of the answers to living well and longer lie within our minds. It's all about perspective and perception. This book is about all the ways you get to control your reaction.

I'm a straight shooter. If you really want to be the best you can be at whatever your age is right now, you must look in the mirror of truth about your own misconceptions. To get what you want, you need to identify what you don't want. When asked how he sculped the famous statue of David, Michelangelo replied, "I just got rid of everything that wasn't David."

Gerontologist Alex Comfort claimed that what we consider "aging" is only 25 percent the result of actual changes in body and mind; the rest is caused by the negative stereotypes placed on older folks. That's what my well-researched message is all about. First, how to recognize and say no to all the ridiculous stereotypes in the media about aging and figure out your own bias. Then to illuminate what your realistic choices are to have the best body, mind, and spirit you can, from now on. Through my personal stories of being in the media and a gathering of the best scientific data, you'll discover your own uniqueness to age gratefully and gracefully. Each chapter ends with Your Turn Now, for you to reflect on the new information and process it into an expanded way of thinking and behaving.

In these pages you will discover the role genetics and environment play in the aging process. Did you know that genetics are just 30 percent responsible in determining how long you live? Behavioral choices are the other 70 percent. (And by the time you hit fifty, lifestyle accounts for 80 percent of how you age!) As my friend Dr. Francis Collins said after his group decoded the human genome, "We're not marionettes being directed by our genes. We have free will to make daily choices."

What Dr. Collins's historic scientific discovery means is that the choices you and I make every day matter the most in how long and well we live. For example, heart disease is the number one cause of death, but 70 percent of arterial aging is preventable. Fifty percent of illnesses associated with aging (diabetes, broken bones, heart attack, and more) can be prevented. You'll learn about the differences between chronological and biological aging and what commonsense choices you can make to be healthier in body, mind, and spirit.

You'll find out the secrets of some of the healthiest old people on the planet—the Okinawans, who are fit and functioning into their nineties and beyond. Doctors who've studied them claim that 80 percent of the nation's coronary units, one-third of the cancer wards, and a lot of the nursing homes would be shut down if Americans made choices more like these elders. And you'll meet several others groups of fabulously long-living folks—a group of nuns, for instance, whose inner lives have been studied for decades, as well as folks who have been tracked by Harvard for over fifty years. They'll point us in the direction of what emotional and spiritual qualities we can begin cultivating and specific behaviors to stay vigorous and become happier throughout our entire existence.

You'll even see why practicing gratitude is so important and how an everyday simple act of being generous can add years to your life.

We'll also address the challenges of caring for parents while we're aging. I'll offer steps to deal with the grief that comes with loss, and explain how to nurture friendships and romantic love through the life span. And of course you'll be hearing from me about what I am learning from my own personal adventure of aging and inside stories of celebrity friends. Since laughter is such a life enhancer, I intend that we have a rollicking good time along the way. (A few birthday party games for when we're older: (1) Sag, You're It; (2) Pin the Toupee on the Bald Guy; (3) Twenty Questions Shouted into Your Good Ear; (4) Hide and Go Pee.)

Ultimately, my fondest hope is that you become inspired to CHANGE: Choose Having A New Growth Experience. This is the only life we get, don't waste another drop. Really, that's the whole point of living, whatever the decade you find yourself in. Grief expert Elisabeth Kübler-Ross put it this way: "It is not the end of the physical body that should worry us. Rather, our concern must be to *live* while we're alive—to release our inner selves from the spiritual death that comes with living behind a facade designed to conform to external definitions of who and what we are."

In order for us to be fulfilled, you and I should begin challenging negative media images that contribute to depression around aging. In many ways, we seventy-eight million baby boomers are already doing that.

# Change That Tune

"Change is the mantra of aging."

—RAM DASS

One thing that's changing is how long we are living—life expectancy for American women is now 90.1 years and for men it's 74.8 years. And every day it increases by seven hours! Evidence shows taking a brisk thirty-minute walk three times a week can add three years to your life. Know what the fastest growing age group in the United States is? Those over hundred—in the 1950s there were just over two hundred folks who reached the century mark; now there are many thousands. There are so many that researchers can now study them as a group. One of the biggest studies is the New England Centenarian Study, which found centenarians (people over one hundred) living "surprisingly productive lives, learning new forms of artistic expression, and waking up each day with eager anticipation," wrote the study's authors in *Living to 100*. That's music to my ears!

Because of scientific understanding of the aging process, we can live much happier, healthier, more vibrant lives than our "parents, grandparents, or anyone else in all of biological time," says internist Henry S. Lodge, coauthor of *Younger Next Year*. I'll point out the right choices so you can look forward to lives of physical strength, mental vigor, and spiritual fullness for decades to come.

Truly Grandma—and Grandpa—aren't what they used to be. And we're showing the next generation new images of aging. Cards from our grandkids Gracie and Elijah decorate my husband Larry's office. They've drawn pictures of him pumping iron with captions like, "U Rock, Papaw!"

Sociologists John and Mathilda Reilly say that we used to think of education as the activity of youth, work as the task of midlife, and leisure as the activity of aging. This idea, they claim, was created at the beginning of the twentieth century, when the average life expectancy was forty-seven. As we live longer, what appears to be evolving is a model in which you and I actually need to have education, work, and leisure throughout our entire lives.

The more you and I continue to learn, to contribute meaningfully to society, and to have time for pleasurable pursuits, the more we will enjoy our lives no matter the length. This, say the Reillys, is much more the way women have lived their lives in the past. That doesn't surprise me.

Baby boomers have revolutionized and remodeled so many aspects of society in the last thirty years. From taking reproductive control—now men can be in the delivery room—to being in sports and becoming CEOs, women are breaking all sorts of other barriers. That's not to say that there isn't still work to be done, but we've already witnessed huge cultural shifts. I want more!

This is the next big cultural shift—redefining aging—and I believe women like us will again lead the way. Author Gail Sheehy, famous for her book *Passages*, suggests we rename the period between sixty and eighty the "Age of Mastery" or the "Second Adulthood." Studies show that men and women are more hopeful about the future and feel happier about getting older than we expected. We're confident about our ability to cope and are excited about what this next phase will bring. (A recent bumper sticker on a cherry red Corvette: "I'm still hot—it just comes in flashes now.") You and I will actualize the dreams we shelved in the first half of our lives to raise families. For instance, full-time college enrollment by older women is up 31 percent in the past ten years. We have a powerful urge to help others and to talk about what we're learning with others.

Any time I see an older woman—whether it's at the drugstore or walking down the street—radiating that sense of a fully blossomed wise being, I try to acknowledge her. Let's begin recognizing and appreciating those who are showing us the way.

I've had several wonderful women as my aging gratefully mentors. Growing up in Kentucky, I was around strong, independent Appalachian women who gave birth to their babies at home, and put in a complete garden, and canned for the winter into their seventies. They didn't worry about their looks—they simply pulled their hair back and got on with it. Minnie Yancey in Berea, Kentucky, can shear a sheep, card and spin the wool, then weave it on a loom she built. Oh, and she can do it wearing combat boots!

A public figure celebrated for her class and aging gratefully is Candice Bergen. I liked her the minute we met. When quizzed in *Ladies' Home Journal* about being sixty, she responded, "Except for the dying part, getting older is so fabulous. I love it. . . . Everybody I know is better older. They're more relaxed, they're more mellow, they're more alert as a friend, they have a confidence. . . . You really do acquire a kind of 'I don't give a damn' about what people think, which is so liberating. I love this age now."

My mom is my survivor mentor. The first time I really saw that was in my teens when my brother Brian died. As devastated and obliterated as she was, Mom clung to a sense of "I've got three other children and a husband now, and they need to eat. They're hungry right now. Their school clothes need washing." Later, when my dad left her for a younger woman and she had to support herself, she dug deep to survive. She identified her marketable skill and became a cook on a riverboat. She then married the captain. Living well is the best revenge.

In her seventies, Mom started going to city commissioner meetings because she always cared about our hometown. The next thing anybody knew, she said, "Hey, I know as much about this city as anybody else," and campaigned for a seat. She won. It was one of the busiest and happiest phases of her life. Mom used her beliefs and values to figure out that one of her passions is serving others. Today, at seventy-eight, she tools around town in her canary yellow BMW convertible, blasting Aretha Franklin.

Another aging mentor was Ms. Jennie Grant. She was the infamous ringleader of a group of five ladies who met at Choice's Restaurant on Main Street in my hometown of Franklin, Tennessee, after church every Sunday. They were always dressed to the nines. The first time I met them I declared, "Are these the former Miss Americas?" Ms. Jennie was a widow with a dowager's hump who walked with a cane. Her distinctive cackling laugh announced her entrance the minute she strolled into a room. She would wave that cane in the air and holler, "I'm still here and raising cane." Wy, Ashley, and I were so drawn to her that we began visiting her at her home, and when she moved into a nursing home, we had her over for supper.

She taught us a cheer from her reign as the first cheerleader in Franklin. Piggly Wiggly and H.G. Hill grocery stores sponsored the football team, so the cheer goes: "Acka packa piggly wiggly h.g. hill, who's gonna win, Ashley will [or Wy, or you]." Wynonna, Ashley, and I remember and honor Ms. Jennie's youthful exuberance anytime we're getting ready to perform live or start a new movie. Do you have older friends?

There are all kinds of other examples of vibrant aging in our culture. Think of George H. W. Bush, who is still skydiving at eighty-one. Or former astronaut John Glenn, who returned to space at seventy-seven to help NASA do studies of bone loss and sleep in aging.

Consider Mary Fasano, who left school at age fourteen to work in a cotton mill, promising herself that she would return to school one day.

As so often happens, work and raising five children got in the way. Ignoring popular opinion, at age seventy-one, she started college. At age eighty-nine, she graduated from Harvard University, having earned honors grades in math, foreign languages, philosophy, and literature. My own mom, Mary, and millions of others like her are proudly announcing the good news about aging. Gratefully.

I loudly proclaim my age to do my part to help people get over the ridiculous stigma about getting older. Whatever your age—start saying it loud and proud. Like Gandhi advised, we must be the change we want to see in the world.

## The Gifts of Aging

"You only perceive real beauty in a person as they get older."
—ANOUK AIMEE

Getting older means organic decay—starting at age twenty, we lose millions of brain cells a year; at some point our hair begins to turn white, our skin sags and wrinkles. You can paint things. You can patch and prop them up. You can fool Mother Nature temporarily, but eventually Father Time is going to cause signs of entropy. That's reality, and I believe it's important to embrace reality.

But while there are some physical losses that come with age, there are far more benefits! Benefits of the heart and spirit that can come only with experience and wisdom. When we focus on those, losing thin thighs or a twenty-inch waist don't seem so important. For instance, studies of older people reveal that by middle age, wounds of childhood don't affect us as much. And as people get older, the majority actually becomes *more* mentally healthy—more forgiving, more cheerful in the face of hardship, and less prone to anger. We're not just growing older, we're growing better!

I am much more comfortable in my own skin now than when I was young. There are so many pictures of my twenty years in show business, and I'm struck by how I slathered on the makeup. What was I thinking? All that time and effort spent, let alone the obvious fact that too much makeup detracts from our essence. Now it's easier to accept myself as I am. I now use makeup to enhance rather than cover up who I am and what I look like. I also have more free time.

At a gig with Dolly Parton, I asked her how long it takes her to get ready. "I can do the whole thing top to bottom in an hour," she chirped. I was surprised. "Well," she then said, "you know, I'm not there when they do my hair." Her most famous line? "You'd be surprised how much it costs to look this cheap." It's now part of her image, but she's also gained a lot of wisdom in her life. My favorite Dolly saying? "Find out who you are and do it on purpose." Amen, sister.

That's one of the greatest gifts of aging I've discovered—the willingness to be wholeheartedly myself. To say and do what I please, with no apologies. I try—and I've raised Wy and Ashley—to be defined from within and speak their own truth. Of course it sometimes comes back to bite me on the butt. In our twenties and thirties, we waste precious minutes, hours, days, and years being concerned about what others are saying and thinking about us. In our forties and fifties, we have so many questions about what's going on that we're just not so concerned about other folks' opinions. And when we hit sixty, we realize they weren't thinking or looking at us at all—they were too busy being concerned about themselves. (Socialite Brooke Astor, at the age of ninety-two, said, "When I was forty, I used to wonder what people thought of me. Now I wonder what *I* think of them.")

If I knew then what I know now, I certainly would not have

wasted so much time worrying about everyone else's opinions of me. And if that's how you're spending your time, maybe the fact that I'm sharing this with you right now can cut down on future wasted time. I certainly hope so. As a hope seller, I'm here to sell you on yourself. I want you to buy into your own potential to be your very best. That means shutting down worrying about what anyone else thinks. Instead of "Hey, look at me," you'll pause to check in with yourself and ask, "Why am I doing this?"

How much more enjoyable would today suddenly become if you let go of the expectations of others? Since I've given up the "disease to please," I don't have the tension and the pressure. The contentment parlays back into fewer wrinkles since you're not scrunched up frowning. Happiness is the best cosmetic. And that gets back to the word *whole.* I feel whole. I'm in control of my day. I don't do stuff if I don't want to. My life is not perfect, but it's full.

In her book *Plan B,* best-selling author Anne Lamott writes about going to a wedding and being surrounded by young women. Instead of being envious, she smiles secretly to herself, delighted to be fifty-something. She writes, "I know many of the women who were at the wedding fear getting older, and I wish I could gather them together, and give them my word of honor that every one of my friends loves being older, loves being in her forties, fifties, sixties, seventies. . . . Look, my feet hurt some mornings, and my body is less forgiving when I exercise. . . . But I love my life more, and me more. I'm so much juicer. And as that old saying goes, it's not that I think less of myself, but I think of myself less often. And that feels like heaven to me."

As a celebrity, in a few superficial ways my life may be a tad easier than yours. But the advantages from the passing years are available to anyone. My friend Nina Chodniewicz and I were chatting after church about aging. She began to laugh. "I am now in my fifties and feel and look better than I did in my thirties. In my thirties I was overwhelmed by the responsibilities of raising seven children," she explained. "Recently, my husband and I were looking at home movies of when I was in my thirties running after all those kids. My husband stared at the images of me in shock. 'You looked like an old Ukrainian peasant then,' he commented. 'You look much younger now.' And it's true. I finally have time for me. And the dessert? All my children and my husband of thirty-four years feel so bad about how worn out I was then that now they pamper me and treat me like a queen."

Probably the best gift is perspective. I call on my frame of reference whenever the need arises. I remember that I am a survivor and then put to use what I've learned. After a quarter century of living, learning, and growing together, my relationship with Larry is better than it has ever been. We're together 24/7. I mean literally. If he goes out to the barn to feed the cows or barn cats or goes to town to pick up feed, that's practically the only time we're apart. He has poker nights, plays golf, and loves to fish with his buddies. We've worked out our stuff. Our lives are so much more peaceful, so harmonious. We can relax into it instead of having to work at it really hard.

Eleven years ago in the issue of *People* on celebrities turning fifty, I acknowledged that "My clock has always been askew. A wife and mother at 18, college degree in my 30s, major career at 37. I may join a SWAT team when I hit 60." I'm now putting the SWAT thing off until I'm eighty.

I hope you can see some of your issues in my journey, because I sure as heck see myself in you. As you may have figured out by now, this book is not "anti-aging." That term connotes wasting time and effort fighting the inevitable. My message here is about finding yourself, discovering your unique beauty inside and out. My goal is to share my secrets of how to become comfortable with your physical appearance as well as embrace the exciting emotional and spiritual possibilities of this life stage so that you actually enjoy aging. When you feel better on the inside, it will become visible to others looking at the outside. You won't feel like you have to fake it, buy it, borrow it, lose it, ignore it.

# Your Turn Now

- This book will inform you with many choices. One idea can change your life. If you open your mind and heart to these ideas, it will help transform the next part of your life. To have a happy, healthy life, you need to face what's standing in your way now and deal with it so that you can enjoy your second half. That's why I've included this quiz here. It will help you understand where you might need to do some work. That way the rest of the book can be as useful to you as possible.

## ARE YOU AGING GRACEFULLY?

1. *When someone starts talking about the latest hot twenty-four-year-old TV star, I*

A. can give an exact time line of all her major hookups and breakups.

B. might have an opinion on her new beau, hairstyle, or project.

C. could care less.

The best answer is C. Even though I'm in the entertainment industry. I think it's very important not to buy into the media's obsession with youth. Studies show that television watching increases women's discontent with their bodies and increases negative ideas about aging. And no wonder—since you hardly ever see a woman over forty on TV. (For more on how the media's youth obsession is damaging to your health and what you can do about it, see Chapter 2.)

**2.** *True or false: Doing absolutely nothing on a regular basis is good for your mind, body, and spirit.*

True. Stress ages the body, which is why it's essential to carve out time to relax and recharge. Spending time alone with no cell phones, computers, or other distractions calms both mind and body, and enables you to focus on what matters most in your life. (For more on how to simplify and destress your life, see Chapter 3.)

**3.** *The best thing about my job is that it*

    A. helps me provide for my family.

    B. gets me out of the house and interacting with others.

    C. puts my talents to good use.

The best answer is C. Studies show that people who are passionate about their work have lower levels of stress and depression, and live longer. While not everyone is lucky enough to have a job that she loves, everyone can find ways to use her talents and bring meaning to her life, which is the tonic that keeps us healthy and vibrant. (For more information, see Chapter 4.)

**4.** *On my birthday, I usually feel*

A. great. The older I get, the wiser and more aware I am of what's good in my life.

B. terrible. I think about all the things that aging takes away from me, like my girlish figure and my ability to rock-climb.

C. Birthday? Darling, I haven't had a birthday in years.

The best answer is A. Most Americans think of aging in terms of the negatives. We worry about losing our looks, strength, and independence. We'd be so much better off if we focused on the positive aspects of aging, like gaining a healthier perspective on life and a deeper spirituality. Not only will we feel better about getting older, having a sunnier outlook can actually keep us healthier. Studies have shown that people with a positive attitude have a reduced risk for Alzheimer's disease, heart disease, diabetes, high blood pressure, and premature death. (For more on cultivating healthier attitudes on aging—and everything else—see Chapter 5.)

**5.** *When I'm sick, I*

A. usually take care of myself. I'm very independent and don't believe in bothering others, especially when I'm unwell.

B. recruit my husband or close friends to bring me soup and romantic comedies.

C. pop some vitamin C and get on with my day. Sick is as sick does.

The best answer is B. A Swedish study found that people with the fewest social ties die younger than those who have a strong support network. Other studies confirm that people with close friends and/or relatives are healthier and happier, and get fewer colds. (See Chapter 6 for more information on how to build your support network.)

**6.** *If one of my children told me he or she had just been accepted to a prestigious law school, I'd be most likely to say,*

A. "Congratulations! I'm so thrilled that you've found your calling."

B. "Are you sure you want to be a lawyer? Law school is very expensive, so I hope you'll think long and hard before taking out all those student loans."

C. "I hope it's nearby. It would be so hard for me if you lived all the way across the country."

The best answer is A. Having a good relationship with your family is essential to aging gracefully, and one of the best ways to do that is to have good communication skills. When someone gives you good news, it's important to acknowledge and celebrate the accomplishment—and not to inflict your own agenda. If you have reservations, you can bring them up gently, at a later date. (For more information on developing a healthy relationship with relatives, see Chapter 7.)

**7.** *I try to keep my weight under control by:*

    A. dieting. I like to have a strict plan.

    B. eating what I really want but in small amounts.

    C. checking the scale every day.

The best answer is B. Excess weight is associated with increased risk for high blood pressure, high cholesterol, diabetes, heart attack, stroke, and other serious illnesses. It also makes you feel more fatigued and look older. So it's important to keep your weight down. But weighing yourself every morning will only drive you crazy—and set a bad tone for the day when you're not happy with your number. Strict diets usually lead to frustration and deprivation and, ultimately, cheating. That's why I agree with Mireille Guiliano. author of *French Women Don't Get Fat:* Eat what you like, but in small portions. It's also important to savor your food, rather than eating a bowl of pasta in front of the TV. When you really allow yourself to fully experience the taste, smell, and texture of your meals, you'll find you can actually feel more satisfied even when you eat less. (For more of my tips on staying fit physically, see Chapter 8.)

**8.** *True or false: Set routines are good for you because your brain doesn't have to work so hard.*

False. Routines are comfortable, but research shows that the brain needs to be constantly learning something new or else it begins to deteriorate. (For more information on mind fitness, see Chapter 8.)

**9.** *True or False: I've updated my wardrobe in the past five years.*

True. While you don't ever want to dress like a teenager, part of aging gracefully is keeping your wardrobe current with the times. (See Chapter 9 for other tips on looking good—as well as some very important fashion no-nos.)

**10.** *When I think of my own death, I*

> A. have it all mapped out, from my will to my "do not resuscitate" orders to the Bible readings at my funeral.

> B. am terrified.

> C. don't think about death. I think about today!

The best answer is A. We're all going to die one day, and though it may seem frightening, facing this fact is one of the most empowering things that you can do. Because I have faith in God, I don't see death as a bad thing and have planned for the same way I do my retirement or my Christmas shopping. (For more information on developing a spiritual life and a healthy relationship with mortality, see Chapter 10.)

Sit down with a pen and piece of paper or at your computer and write the answers to the following questions.

- When you think of aging, what images come into your mind? What feelings? What do you look forward to? What are you afraid of?

- Do you make disparaging comments to friends on their birthdays?

- What things do you not do or try because you are "too old"? What would you do right now in your life if your age were not an issue? As famous baseball player Satchel Paige asked, "How old would you be if you didn't know how old you were?"

- How did your parents feel about aging? Who is your role model for the kind of old person you wish to be? What qualities does he or she have that you'd like to cultivate?

- What does aging well mean to you? What are the factors that you believe will contribute to your aging gratefully?

- Identify two positive things about aging. What are the gifts of aging you've experienced so far?

"Hollywood is a place where they'll pay you 50,000 dollars for a kiss and 50 cents for your soul."

—MARILYN MONROE

# 2 | *Star Wars:* Using Your Central Intelligence in Winning the Aging Culture War

WOMEN OF MANY OTHER NATIONS are oppressed by regimes that won't allow them first-class citizenship, careers, or even an education. So why is it that American women imprison themselves in their own inferiority complexes about weight, body image, and fashion? Ninety percent of us are unhappy with our bodies. Yes, we can go to college, but a sizable number of American female students has an eating disorder, despite the education. We've made so many important legal, economic, and social advances and yet we're unable to let go of unrealistic expectations of physical beauty. I call it voluntary misery. We're hypnotized by impossible ideals. But we can snap out of it.

The first time I didn't get a job in the media because of my age, I went to my bedroom, shut the door, and confronted myself. "Uh-oh, Miss Smarty, Miss Aging Gratefully. So how are you feeling now?" Several reactions made me hyper. First of all, I hadn't even been aware I was up for the TV role. My TV agent at William Morris, Krista Parkinson, reported that everyone at the network felt I was perfect. However, one guy suggested that they "go younger." Long ago I became convinced that Hollywood is out of touch with the rest of America, but now it was personal. I felt victimized.

As a justice fighter, I was so angry for all of us. Since I'm the mother of two daughters who work in this industry, I called Wy and Ash to vent. They were instantly incredulous. Ashley, my activist feminist, insisted I report the incident in this book and talk about it every chance I get. Wy wanted to "pinch the idiot on the underside of his upper arm." But I'm guessing it also made them less secure in their own careers, so I felt protective. I flashed on Colin Powell's words to me: "Good ideas don't become reality unless they have a champion."

## Ready for Prime Time

Sometimes man's rejection is God's protection. That same week I was offered my own show on the Hallmark Channel. On *Naomi's New Morning,* one of the topics we discuss is how to figure out who you really are and then live more fully. Star Jones Reynolds from *The View* was one of the first guests and made this statement about weight, age, and appearance: "You must be the only dictionary that defines you."

Fortunately one of the gifts of aging is that I no longer take rejection personally. Having spent decades in and around showbiz, it's so obvious that very few actors are lucky enough to have a career after the age of forty. Studios and producers practice discrimination against mature actors because they erroneously believe that the best target consumer demographic is eighteen- to thirty-four-year-olds.

So many women get terrified, angry, or envious. Some, like Joan Rivers, have had so much plastic surgery that only one side of their face moves. Priscilla Presley and Kenny Rogers don't even look like themselves anymore. Many stars are rumored to use human growth hormone to keep their youthful appearance, which could possibly increase the risk of diabetes, liver and kidney problems, and cancers such as breast, prostate, and colon. Being an entertainer, that could have been me if I hadn't figured out its insanity. But I realized years ago that to survive in showbiz, I had to have an attitude adjustment rather than constant cosmetic interventions. I've had an "about-face" on this issue.

I'm using this book as a bullhorn to expose the harm of pop culture's stereotyping against aging. The media's ill-placed obsession with youth and beauty is seriously hurting people of all ages.

In many ways, I'm in an interesting position. Although for my whole life people have said I'm pretty, it has only made me more aware of beauty's unimportance. My looks may have helped my career, but they have not brought me happiness. Happiness has come from witnessing the impact of human kindness—being kind to myself and others, focusing on the positive, laughing at myself. In therapy, I've come to see the necessity of healing my wounds from the past, copping to my mistakes, and taking responsibility for more healthy choices in the here and now. I've done what I can to develop healthy self-esteem and learn to live from the inside out. These inner qualities, I've discovered, bring more joy and peace than any set of perfect lips, flawless skin, or mass of hair. Life is not a beauty contest. But that's not the message we're exposed to day in and day out. (What was the most requested nose of 2005? Nicole Kidman's, say plastic surgeons.) "Politically I'm a hypocrite," says Brett Butler. "I'm a socialist with a gold card. I think we need a revolution but I'm scared I won't be able to find any good moisturizer after it happens."

A beautiful woman is an accident of nature. A beautiful older woman is a work of grace and character. The poetry of nature. After thirty, you are responsible for your own face. And what's happening on the inside does indeed start showing on the outside.


# Where Have All the Older Women Gone?

"A man's as old as he's feeling. A woman as old as she looks."
—MORTIMER COLLINS

It's older women who suffer the most from media age bias. Recently I met Sally Field, who also turned sixty last year. She looks great! When I told Sally about this book, she confided a disturbing experience. Her clothes stylist brought a bunch of outfits to try on but reported that one designer refused to loan out clothes to her because Sally was "too old." "I grew up in the fifties," she confided in me. "I couldn't let my feelings out back then. The stage [acting] allows me to see what the world looks like through others' eyes. These experiences have broadened my insights; now I am more confident and appreciate what all the years have taught me."

The Screen Actors Guild reported a couple of years ago that only 24 percent of all women's roles on prime-time TV went to women over forty. When Kim Cattrall accepted a Golden Globe for *Sex and the City,* she revealed that the day she hit forty, the number of roles she was up for reduced by half.

The movie world is similar. Joan Chen took a four-year break from acting when she was forty. When she returned, she confided, filmmakers saw her very differently: "I used to be their dream lover. Now I'm their dream mother." Even Oscar-winning actors like Sissy Spacek and Meryl Streep decry the lack of roles for middle-aged women. And guess who gets the Oscar statuette most often? Older men and younger women. "Half of Hollywood is worried they'll be perceived as too old for their next job and the other half should be," said one agent. Jodie Foster admits that the realities of Hollywood prompted a midlife crisis: "Eighty percent of movies written for women I can't get, and I have to find something good out of the remaining 20 percent. . . . I keep thinking like, oh, I guess it's over."

Nowhere does ageism show up more boldly than in the May-December pairings we see all the time on the big screen. Lauren Bacall was nineteen when she was teamed in *To Have and Have Not* with forty-five-year-old Humphrey Bogart. Sophia Loren was thirty-three years younger than Clark Gable in *It Started in Naples*. In the nineties, there was a slew of such pairings: Harrison Ford, in his fifties, with Anne Heche, thirties; Jack Nicholson, sixties, with Helen Hunt, thirties; Robert Redford, sixties, with Kristin Scott Thomas, thirties. These movies convey the message that men are sexy at any age, but women should go around with bags on their heads after hitting forty.

There have been a few movies that reverse the pairing—*How Stella Got Her Groove Back*, with forty-something Angela Bassett teamed with twenty-something Taye Diggs, or the famous "Mrs. Robinson" from *The Graduate* come to mind. In these movies, one of the plotlines is the age difference, which is something that never gets mentioned when the situation is reversed. Demi Moore and Ashton Kutcher grab headlines, most of which emphasize the age difference. Despite all the changes women have initiated over the past thirty years in work and family life, the media continues to reinforce the erroneous idea that a woman is vital and worthwhile only if she is young and beautiful.

This idea is not only unfair to women of a certain age; it is robbing our girls of a normal childhood. They have shorter childhoods and then take much longer to grow up and mature. Ironically, they will also have longer life spans. Advertisers promote precocious dressing—Target and JCPenney now sell thong underwear to grade schoolers. Anorexia, bulimia, depression, and even suicide are all too common with teens. Experts estimate that 5 out of every 100 young women are bingeing and purging or starving themselves to death. Girls read magazines that tell them how to seduce a guy and offer dieting tips, while looking at images of impossibly gorgeous models and actresses. No wonder their young and impressionable minds despair about measuring up.

In some ways, it's a terrible illusion that's causing such suffering—even the most gorgeous women don't look perfect in real life. Here's a dose of reality from the December 1990 issue of *Esquire* magazine. An invoice for touching up a photo of Michelle Pfeiffer (who was all of thirty-three years old at the time) reads: "Clean up complexion, soften eye lines, soften smile line, add color to lips, trim chin, remove neck lines, soften line under ear lobe, add highlights to earrings, add blush to cheek, clean up neck line, remove stray hair, remove hair strands from dress, adjust color and add hair on top of head . . ." If Michelle Pfeiffer needs this much of a touch-up, *no one* can live up to the ideal.

(This reminds me of a joke. How many members of a star's entourage does it take to change a lightbulb? Eight: one to apologize for it being out; one to investigate the best type of replacement; one to do the makeup, hair, and wardrobe; one to test, then hold the ladder; one to direct; one to relate the experience to the media; one to take photos; and one to do touch-ups.)

Even the world's most beautiful women don't feel they measure up. In a photo book a famous photographer did years ago on famous beauties, every one of those women spoke only of her flaws. It's time for all of us to break free of the beauty myths imposed on us to sell products and embrace our inner beauty—whatever our age.

## What You See Is Not What You'll Get

"For the first time in human history, most of the stories are told to most of the children, not by their parents, their school, or their church but by a group of distant corporations that have something to sell. This unprecedented condition has a profound effect on the way we are socialized into our roles, including age as a social role."
—GEORGE GERBNER, WRITING ABOUT THE POWER
OF THE MEDIA

Researchers tell us that older people suffer from more negative stereotyping than any other social group, and that the media are one of the main contributing factors to such prejudice. Studies show that, while the number of old people is continuing to rise, they are underrepresented in TV and movies, with—surprise!—older women being the most underrepresented. In one study of 464 roles on prime-time TV, only 1.5 percent was for women over sixty-four. When older folks do appear, they tend to be shown as feeble-minded, stubborn, or helpless, objects to avoid or make fun of. Through these powerful messages, we are taught to fear getting older and to expect the worst from this natural process.

Negative notions of aging are so widespread that when former president Jimmy Carter mentioned that he was writing his book *The Virtues of Aging*, most people responded, he claimed, by saying, "Virtues?

What could possibly be good about growing older?" They need this book!

Even common language reflects our prejudice. Have you ever noticed that when we're young, we can't wait to get older? I'm five and a half, we proudly tell everyone in sight. In our teens, we exaggerate up— *almost* sixteen we say, often from thirteen onward. And what's the day we all long for? The day we *become* twenty-one. Then it's all downhill from there: We *turn* thirty (like milk spoiling). We're *pushing* forty, fifty, sixty, seventy, eighty, as if the weight of our years is rocks we must carry in front of us. Then we're *over the hill. Put out to pasture.*

And what about all those birthday cards that bemoan growing older? One study found that 39 percent of greeting cards dealt with aging negatively, although humorously. And a study of jokes in general found that aging jokes deal almost exclusively with the decline of sexual ability and interest, mental functioning, or death. Fun stuff, huh?

Doris Roberts, feisty costar of *Everyone Loves Raymond,* took on the media a few years ago when testifying before the Senate Special Committee on Aging. "My peers and I are portrayed as dependent, helpless, unproductive, and demanding rather than deserving. This is not just a sad situation. . . . It's a crime," she declared. And the crime is that such portrayals are far from the truth. As seventy-one-year-old Doris went on to say: "I'm at the peak of my life. When my children say I rock, they're not talking about a rocking chair." As my friend George Jones sang in his hit song, "I Don't Need No Rockin' Chair."

Our children are being raised by electronic appliances that bombard them with these attitudes. Young people age eight to eighteen are now spending an average of six and a half hours a day "plugged in": watching TV and videos, listening to music, or being online. Sixty-eight percent have a TV in their bedroom, and they watch ninety more minutes of television a day and do less reading and homework than those who don't. About 50 percent have no rules about what they can watch or for how long.

Except for *7th Heaven,* not since *The Andy Griffith Show* have I seen a show on TV that portrayed a parent as an intelligent human being. On many of the shows, viewers are taught that adults are bumbling idiots, and their instructions are to be ignored. One study found that if older people are shown at all in children's cartoon programs, they're either evil characters or weaklings in need of the superhero's help. All of these ridiculous portrayals are a major reason why the elderly in our society are mocked and disrespected.

There's ageism behind the camera as well. A talk show in Chicago made news when it was revealed that it screened out any person whose voice sounded "old."

Susan Taggart wrote in a brave article in *Focus Over Fifty* about "a pronounced age prejudice in Hollywood. They look at most writers over the age of 35 as unemployable." To get work, she claims, older writers now go so far as to hire youngsters to pretend they've written their script so that it will be seriously considered.

It's the same story in commercials. Remember that awful Lay's Potato Chip commercial in which apparently feebleminded and decrepit grandparents tussled over a bag of chips? One researcher discovered that advertising executives prefer to market to people their own age, thirty- to thirty-nine-year-olds, with twenty-somethings coming in second—in both preferred markets and age of ad executives. It's a self-fulfilling prophecy—appeal only to young people and only young people'll buy your products.

The reason advertisers ignore us, they say, is that middle-aged and older Americans are loyal to certain brands so advertising is wasted on them. Not so, says a study done by the AARP—folks over forty-five are just as likely as younger people to switch brands and try new products.

So there! Consumer advocate Ralph Nader once told me, "It takes a bit of a civic personality and a mature mind to put human value over commerciality."

Wake up and smell the demographics! as the head of the American Society of Aging once said. Right now, the over-fifty crowd makes up only 26 percent of the 300 million U.S. population, but we account for 20 percent of total U.S. spending. And we're reaching the big 5-0 at the rate of one person every seven seconds! By 2020, Americans fifty and older will be 36 percent of the population. And this group of baby boomers controls 70 percent of this country's wealth. Ignoring us makes no economic sense at all.

## Why the Media Matters

"The biases the media has are much bigger than conservative or liberal. They're about getting ratings, about making money, about doing stories that are easy to cover."

—AL FRANKEN

Why do I get so passionate when I talk about this unjust state of affairs? Why should it matter that older people are invisible or portrayed negatively in the media? It matters for many important reasons. It's priming our next generation for emotional problems. Plus, research has shown that negative images of aging may actually significantly decrease your life span. A study done at Yale that looked at such beliefs as "When you get old, you're worthless" found that older people with more negative perceptions of aging lived an average of 7.5 years less than those with positive ones. That's a huge difference.

Health alert: How you feel about getting older has a greater effect on how long you will live than having low blood pressure or low cholesterol (which are associated with a four-year increase) or having lower body fat, not smoking, and exercising regularly (which have been found to add one to three years to your life). See why we must dismantle the cultural bias against aging! It is literally killing us. How about paying attention to numbers like your cholesterol and triglycerides before your scale weight?

Since television was invented, a debate has been raging over whether its violence, sexual content, ageism, etc., has a negative impact on our society, particularly children. Folks on the business side claim that TV is merely a reflection of who we are, rather than an active force in shaping us.

That's why I was so interested to learn about the Buddhist kingdom of Bhutan, an isolated nation in the Himalayas that claims to be interested in GNH (gross national happiness) rather than GNP (gross national product). In 1999, its ruler lifted a ban on television. Suddenly they went from nothing to forty-six channels. Take a guess what happened. An immediate and sharp upsurge of crime, drug use, and divorce. School violence increased so much that there had to be "marathon staff meetings" to deal with the issue. One-third of parents declared to researchers that they were now more interested in watching the tube than talking with their children.

Studies on a Canadian town where TV was introduced in the seventies show the same increase in violence. And guess what? The more TV you watch, the more you overestimate the wealth of others, the less happy you are, and the fewer sports and social activities you participate in. TV watching has also been shown to increase women's discontent with their bodies and men's discontent with their wives. Scientists have even found that the more TV you watch, the more you hold negative ideas of aging.

The average older person watches forty-three hours of TV a week, the equivalent of a full-time job. When you watch a lot of TV, it not only makes you feel bad about getting older, it makes you restless and less content with your life, no matter your age. You get a false sense not only of what you should look like but also how to create happiness and contentment. The lost hours in front of the tube are hours that are unavailable for self-reflection and connection to others. Do you have the tube on so that you don't have to think?

We are a nation obsessed with celebrities. One reason Americans worship celebrities is that so many of our own families are fractured and scattered. We think of stars as friends or family. We often know more about them than we do of actual relatives. Instead of being a couch potato watching other people on TV, I prefer being out in the real world, watching and relating to real folks. That's why I accept speaking gigs in all fifty states. Last month, I got to hang with folks in Omaha, Nebraska; Naples, Florida; Washington, DC; Dayton, Ohio; Buffalo Gap, Texas; and Lexington, Kentucky.

You can reclaim the rest of your future from the unreal world of pop culture and celebrity worship. Be conscious of the kind of media you support and consume. I recently was offered a lot of money to write a column for *The National Enquirer*. I turned them down flat.

Other cultures revere the wisdom and experience of aging and have realistic standards of what's healthy and attractive. In Okinawa, respect for aging is one of the reasons these people tend to be the world's longest-lived. Elders take enormous pride in their status. Aging is seen as the process of gathering wisdom, something to be honored and celebrated. They have various rites of passage, corresponding to the Chinese zodiac, which occur at ages seventy-three, seventy-eight, eighty-five, eighty-eight, ninety-seven, and one hundred. In these ceremonies, the elder is driven around in a convertible and strangers line the streets to cheer, for it is believed that participating in the ceremony will allow you to share in that person's health, good fortune, and long life. The way they live every day prevents obesity, high blood pressure, thin bones, etc. But their easygoing personalities create what biogerontologists term a "stress-resistant personality." In case you don't know, 85 percent of all illnesses are stress related.

In Japan, wrinkles and gray hair are considered signs of wisdom. Elders have prestige; there's even a Japanese national holiday called Honor the Aged Day. In the Andes, people even exaggerate their age to gain greater respect. Native Americans historically have seen their elders as "the keepers of wisdom" who protect the tribe with their knowledge and skills. In India, those who follow Hinduism believe that elders have important jobs and can be of service to the community. In ancient Rome the elder citizens filled the most critical roles in society. The Latin word *senex*, meaning "old man," is the root of *senate* and *senior*.

In his book *Still Here*, Ram Dass tells a story about visiting a friend in India. "You're looking so old! . . . You're so gray!" his friend exclaimed. Ram Dass responded with dismay until he realized that the man meant it as the most sincere compliment. He was saying, "How wonderful that you've arrived at old age."

One of my inspirations for this book project was a God Wink, an unexpected insight into a larger truth. At the grocery store I complimented a lovely eighty-year-old woman who obviously took care of herself. She teared up. She was so pleased and surprised by the acknowledgment. That was quite a difference from my experience with an older clerk in a hotel gift shop a week later. We fell into a conversation and the clerk ended up speaking intimately about her life—about coming to the United States fifty years before, the death of her husband, her recent hospitalization, the pros and cons of her job. When I asked, "How old are you, anyway?" she snapped, "That is a rude question." She could reveal everything except the "dirty secret" of her age. I'll be sending her a copy of this book with this page earmarked.

We've become youth worshippers only in the past seventy years or so. Until the nineteenth century, old age was respected in Western culture because it was so rare. Even in 1900, life expectancy in the United States was only forty-seven! The tide began to turn during the Depression when older people were considered burdens because they were seen as taking jobs from younger folks. Since then, we have become more and more obsessed with turning back the clock.

It's a drip-drip effect eroding our self-esteem. Negative stereotypes of aging create a deep fear of growing older. But FEAR is False Evidence Appearing Real. It's not true that aging means a steady decline of physical and mental functioning. It is true, however, that we need meaningful activities and relationships. When we keep our mind/body/spirit engaged, this stage can truly be the most rewarding and interesting of our lives!

Our beliefs will become our biology. We're exposed to hundreds of negative stereotypes a day. We think we are going to decline, and so we do. Here's one example. In an experiment, a researcher at Harvard first reminded older subjects of the benefits of aging—wisdom, greater experience, perspective—and then tested their brain function. Their memories improved. Then she focused on negative stereotypes—that older people are forgetful, for instance—and the same people's memory function dipped down! Words can change brain function.

A group of seventy-five-year-olds were taken to a resort and asked to act for a week as if they were twenty years younger—to think of themselves as still in the middle of their careers, to refer to their children and spouses as if they were twenty years younger, to play music from that era, etc. Guess what? Their memories improved, as did their dexterity, independence, and activity levels. Their hearing, sight, muscle strength, and flexibility got better. And judges comparing "before" and "after" pictures judged them on average to look three years younger than before.

Let's reeducate our brains: Rather than vacuuming the fat out of our thighs, it's time to vacuum out of our brains the out-of-date, death-creating fear of aging that we're incessantly fed by the media.

## Signs of Change

"Don't you wish there were a knob on the TV to turn up the intelligence? There's one marked 'Brightness,' but it doesn't work."

—GALLAGHER

Right now, forty-three million American women are between the ages of forty and sixty. By 2008, we baby boomers will be the largest and richest group not only in the United States, but in the history of the world! Collectively, we have very deep pockets. And unlike women of previous generations, we will have *earned* our money, rather than inherited it. So there.

Obviously, with all these dollars comes real influence—if we choose to use it. Advertisers want these dollars, so now we can vote with our pocketbooks. What products, movies, TV shows, music, and magazines do you want to support? Let's begin using the power of our purses, pocketbooks, and designer bags.

An organization called the Industry Coalition for Age Equality in the Media, founded by Ed Asner and others, is lobbying networks and producers to cast actors over forty, using the buying power of baby boomers as incentives. There are other positive signs of change. My daughter Ashley, thirty-eight, is the spokesperson for Revlon's American Beauty campaign, while Kristin Davis, forty-one, is the new face of Maybelline as of 2006. When she hit the big 4-0, Kristin said, "It's great that actresses that aren't twenty-somethings are being offered contracts by cosmetic companies. Women of all ages are beautiful."

The editor of *Cosmopolitan,* Kate White, runs no articles on crash diets or plastic surgery. "If you are empowering women in their twenties," she says, "why would you give them breast implants?"

I've started to notice lately a few "older" stars on network TV, like Tom Selleck, sixty-one; Candice Bergen, sixty; Betty White, eighty-four; and of course William Shatner, seventy-five. Ashley took me to dinner with Sean Connery and his wife and I was stunned when they both admitted to being seventy-five. When we see Paul Newman at the racetrack (his passion!), I can hardly believe he's eighty-one! Clint Eastwood is seventy-five. And four men in their sixties just appeared on the cover of *Rolling Stone* magazine. Their latest CD has been heralded as their best in twenty years. Can you guess? It's the Rolling Stones.

Hollywood's leading lights are breaking the aging taboo and speaking out about the marvels of maturing. Here are a few of their inspiring voices:

You have to love your smile lines, you have to love your frown lines. . . . Be brave—and be proud not to be like everyone else. —*Nicole Kidman*

I always assumed I wouldn't hit my stride until I was 40. I look back at myself on *Moonlighting* when I had no wrinkles, no character lines or anything. I like the way I look now so much better.—*Bruce Willis*

You get smarter as you get older. And what could be better? Being smarter is better than sex. And there was nothing I liked better than sex.—*Lauren Hutton*

I'm tired of playing worn-out depressing ladies in frayed bathrobes. I'm going to get a new hairdo and look terrific and go back to school and even if nobody notices, I'm going to be the most self-fulfilled lady on the block.—*Joanne Woodward, who left Hollywood in midlife to get a degree at Sarah Lawrence*

I'm so proud that I made it and I'm healthy and strong that I say to all women, "Celebrate your life."—*breast cancer survivor Olivia Newton-John*

[Hollywood has a] barbaric attitude toward older actresses. Having wrinkles is not a reason to be put away. In Europe, they understand that, thank God.—*Charlotte Rampling*

I believe in a sturdy bra with lots of wires and pulleys instead of a boob job.—*Kathy Griffin*

We have a pact that we will never do cosmetic surgery. When we feel weak about Botox or surgery, we'll call each other for support and just say no. Someday we'll be the only two actresses who will get roles for 65-year-old women, because everyone else will look like they're 30.—Téa Leoni speaking of her friendship with Elizabeth Shue

When positive movies on aging appear, they can be very success-ful, which should give Hollywood a big hint. But they still don't get it.

When *Cocoon* came out, 20th Century–Fox banned all publicity photos of "the old people," and focused instead on the grandson. But it was the old people like Jessica Tandy and Hume Cronin whom folks fell in love with and spawned a successful sequel. And remember *On Golden Pond*, as well as the Jessica Tandy character in *Fried Green Tomatoes*?

Films like *Something's Gotta Give* and *Shall We Dance* expose the silliness of May-December pairings and portray age-appropriate mature relationships. What about a *Sex and the City* for sixty-year-olds? Or a *Desperate Housewives* for the post-forties crowd?

Savvy companies are finally getting the message that we have deep pockets and expendable income. The Gap announced the launch of a new clothing chain, Forth and Towne, to cater to women over thirty-five, and JCPenney is starting a line of clothes specifically for over-thirty-five folks. Chico's has been growing like gangbusters with women's clothes for midlife and beyond. *Ladies' Home Journal* has launched a new magazine, *More*, aimed at the over-forty crowd with articles on parenting adult children and other issues of midlife.

Late in 2004, Dove Beauty Bar launched a Campaign for Real Beauty, an attempt to challenge youth-obsessed views of age, beauty, body shape, and race. One of their ads in particular caught my eye—it is of ninety-six-year-old Irene, a beautiful African American, with the text: "Wrinkled? Wonderful? When did beauty become limited by age? It's time to think, talk, and learn how to make beauty real again." Salma Hayek is the most physically beautiful woman I know. But as a family friend, I was first drawn to her personality. She said in an interview, "Beauty projects a sense of well-being and calm, but at the same time it is easiness and stimulation. That's what joy is, and I think that is what beauty is as well, a sensation of calm and excitement at the same time." As I write, she's with Ashley somewhere in Central America for Youth AIDS, where they're drawn to her compassion, not her looks.

Oprah has used her tremendous influence in both her TV show and magazine to promote positive notions of aging. A few years ago, she picked Diane Sawyer and me as role models over fifty. Here's part of what Diane said on the show: "I love my age. . . . You have to start by changing the story you tell yourself about getting older. If you're telling yourself a story about what you are losing and about fear, then that's the story you're going to live. You've just cast yourself in a plot. So the minute you say to yourself that time is everything, and I'm going to make sure that time is used the way I dream it should be used, then you've got a whole different story."

If we had age awards for role models, I'd vote for her.

We all can get out of the media's gravitational pull and help shift the center of cultural gravity. Together, we can usher in a positive view as we're aging.

## Your Turn Now

- What are your stereotypes about old people? Check in with your reactions to those ahead of you chronologically. Name a couple of negative ideas you have. Then challenge yourself to think of people who don't fit the stereotypes.

- Identify a recent media message that made you feel inferior. Too-thin models? No one with wrinkles? In *The Beauty Myth*, Naomi Wolf exposes the way we are all manipulated to feel insecure about our looks in order to create a need for all kinds of products.

- The more you increase your awareness, the less the media will affect you. Become vocal about celebrating your age instead of denying years. You earned them! Say it loud and say it proud: Va va boom!!

- Over fifty? Join the American Association of Retired Persons (AARP). No, you absolutely don't have to be retired.

- See yourself as an aging mentor to those younger than you. Try celebrating your birthday in a happy spirit of real pride. Insist on respect.

- Here's a positive idea from author Victoria Moran: Think of fifty fabulous adjectives to describe yourself right now.

- Do you have any older friends? If not, how might you make some?

- Since the negative messages are so strong, we need each other. Talk about it when you're around your pals. The Red Hat Society comes to mind. This group of women wears purple clothes and red hats when they get together for tea and fun. They have chapters around the country and even national conventions. Here's how the Queen Mother Sue Ellen Cooper describes the origins of the group: "The Red Hat Society began as a result of a few women deciding to greet middle age with verve, humor and élan. We believe silliness is the comedy relief of life, and since we are all in it together, we might as well join red-gloved hands and go for the gusto together." Find out more at www.redhatsociety.com.

- Join the Parents Television Council, whose mission is "to promote and restore responsibility and decency to the entertainment industry in answer to America's demand for positive, family-oriented television programming." In addition to lobbying against sex and violence on TV, they lobby for positive programs depicting elders in a more positive light. Go to www.parentstv.org.

"All my possessions for a moment of time."
—LAST WORDS OF QUEEN ELIZABETH I

# 3 | *Analyze This:* Decluttering Physically, Emotionally, and Spiritually

TO AGE GRATEFULLY, try thinking smaller to live larger. If you hung out with me for a day and night, you'd be surprised to see how I apply this in my home. I wish I could spend time with you and see and hear your priorities as you go about your life.

I've found that as we age, a natural desire emerges to shed things standing in the way of our embracing our genuine selves. Have you been noticing an impulse to pare down, have more time for yourself? Do you crave less stress, more control over your schedule? Do you yearn for simple pleasures, more contentment?

Americans have more leisure time than ever before in history yet complain about never having enough time. Have you ever considered going beyond thinking about this problem and maybe think instead for a moment how you've contributed to it? I'm here to promote and popularize the freedom in simplicity. It's part of my mission statement: to slow down, simplify, and be kind.

I first became aware of the impulse to simplify while touring with Wy. Ever wonder what a touring bus looks like inside? Our mobile home on the road was a forty-foot tour bus. It's a tiny version of a trailer. When you step up, there's a front jump seat similar to a La-Z-Boy recliner. I would relax there after our gig. Wy and Ash called it my throne. It would be two o'clock in the morning. No cell phones back then. I felt like a pioneer woman in a Conestoga wagon setting out across some great frontier.

Behind the jump seat was a minuscule living room with a TV up on the wall and a kitchenette. I'd flop down on the couch with my favorite quilt, a pillow, and my dog Banjo on my belly. Wy and I would make popcorn in the microwave. There was a sink, a built-in coffeemaker, a half-size refrigerator, and a small pantry where we stored staples like canned tuna, peanut butter, and a loaf of bread. There was one bathroom. Beyond that was Wy's bedroom in the middle and mine in the back. In the vanity I kept my hot rollers, makeup, toiletries. A few stage outfits hung in a narrow closet. Family pictures made it feel homey. I called it my womb.

Such tight quarters demanded keeping my stuff to a minimum. I felt a sense of freedom in having so little. I became the lightest packer. Life as a professional hotel guest also reinforced the importance of paring down to bare essentials. A bed, a table with a clock and a Bible in the drawer, a TV, a bathroom, and a window. That's it. In a hotel, you don't have to make your bed or wash the towels, and people even bring you food on a tray! Having cooked and cleaned my whole adult life while also holding down a full-time job and raising two daughters, it was a complete lifestyle switch.

In the quiet of all those thousands of spartan rooms, for the first time in my life, I could sit still and just be. I could listen to my thoughts. Because I wasn't in my kingdom of stuff, I was free to process the new experiences of traveling. Every day I looked out the window on a new scene. I had quiet time to digest what I was discovering about the entertainment world, to think about what was going on in my relationship with Wynonna and Ashley. I didn't have to shop or fix things. I didn't have to rearrange. I didn't have to dust or vacuum. I could get down to what was front and center in my life.

After being away from home, when I returned, the knickknacks stood out. I would look at them with new eyes and realize, "Wait a minute. I don't want this. I don't even like it." Over time, our tastes change. So do our needs. I began to purge my house of everything that I didn't really love. I had seen celebrity mansions, which seemed decorated more for show than for comfort. In today's materialistic culture, celebrities are supposed to reside in humongous estates. But I don't see myself as a celebrity. I'm interested in creating a home, not an image. A psychological fortress. Heaven on earth is enjoying whatever you have. Ease of living and time for family, friends, and just being are my priorities. Recently I was on Martha Stewart's TV show. While cooking together, she asked if my cook was "full-time." I don't have a cook. My friend Dorthey comes three days a week to help out.

My decluttering impulse spread—to cleaning up old issues from my past, relationships that no longer served me, ways of being that were getting in my way. The more I pared down, the better I began to feel.

This is what I'm hoping for you. Psychologists consider our homes a metaphor for our lives. Maybe you still have your mom's couch. A lamp you bought just because it was on sale. Maybe your closets are stuffed with stuff you've outgrown. At some point, as the birthdays pile up, most of us get the urge to step back to look at our lives objectively. It dawns on us that we haven't much time. Every day we pass by chances to let go of junk we don't need—from old clothes to old ways of thinking and acting in our relationships.

Today, did you spend more time wondering about what to eat than how your life is going? Like Queen Elizabeth realized on her deathbed, it hits us that time is our most precious possession. It becomes more urgent with every birthday.

Those "shedding" impulses indicate that you're coming into your own. The young are impulse buyers. It takes maturity to realize that our soul life is more fun and enjoyable than stuff, even cool stuff. Like Sarah Jessica Parker says, "Sometimes I don't shop for a year. There are so many other things to do." Our souls are asking, even demanding, that we begin clearing the way. In the space that opens up, we can begin to design the rest of our future. As we will explore in the next chapter, this stage is all about meaning and purpose.

So come along as we look at how you can lighten up and, as life coach Richard Leider says, "repack your bags" for the rest of your journey.

## Do You Know Enoughness?

"The wise man carries his possessions with him."
—BIAS

If we're to take inventory of our life so far, we must get real and decide whether we're buying too much. Americans use only 20 percent of what they own. The less you have in most cases, the less you have to worry about. Not to mention the money worries buying incurs. Author Judith Levine decided to go a year without shopping. After blowing

$1,000 on holiday gifts and maxing out her credit cards, she decided to not buy anything except bare necessities. In her book *Not Buying It,* she describes how she and her partner had time to talk and hang out, improve their relationship, and have time for themselves.

A friend in her midforties recently downsized with her husband to a condo when their kids left. "I finally realized that my big house and yard was getting in the way of time to myself," she confided. "I had to tell myself the truth—I hate gardening! I am so much happier now to look out onto the lawn knowing it's someone else's problem." When we look clearly at the daily aspects, as this friend did, it's clear what we're holding on to is some fantasy of how our life is supposed to be. Aging is about seeing your life as it really is right now, not how you once thought it would be.

When you finally get around to seeing your truths, maybe you'll discover that it's not the size of your house and yard that needs attention, but what's inside. Maybe you're buried in papers, clogged with kitchen gadgets, or becoming a clotheshorse. Has stuff gathered throughout the house like snowdrifts? If this is something you need help with, you might want to enlist the services of FlyLady. FlyLady (real name Marla Cilley) helps with CHAOS (**C**an't **H**ave **A**nyone **O**ver **S**yndrome) in books and a website (FlyLady.net) with all sorts of helpful hints for taking control of your domestic circumstances. FlyLady breaks down decluttering into tiny steps over a couple months so it won't be overwhelming.

Don't forget your closets. It's easy for them to get filled with dresses from 1984, cool shoes that hurt, purses that someone gave you that you wouldn't be caught dead carrying. Ashley recently called me to help do a big purge. We practiced the two-year rule—if she hadn't worn it in two years, it went. It helped to do it together because if she clung to something I hadn't seen her wear, I helped pry it loose. We have favorite charities we give our clothes to. My friend Reverend Becca Stevens runs

Magdalene House for prostitutes who are in a two-year program to get off the street. For women who are trying to help themselves by going for a job interview, stylish and appropriate clothes can make all the difference. As a single working mom, I once settled for a waitress job at Howard Johnson's because they provided a uniform (it was polyester brown and orange). Dress for Success is another of the places I donate clothing. I've even done benefits for them because I know some of their amazing success stories. Check out Dress for Success when you're looking to make your donations.

After her divorce, Wy had a yard sale to physically and emotionally cleanse herself of everything that could remind her of a very bad marriage. The symbolic gesture filled half an acre and brought in fans from all over. The event was covered by the media and Wy spoke of how "every ending is a new beginning." When asked why I wasn't there, I responded, " 'Cause I gave her a lot of the stuff."

If you'll go through the cleaning-out process, my hunch is that you'll be so freed by the results that soon the whole house, including your wardrobe, will contain only what you use and really love. That's what happened for me. Now, whenever I go in a store, I ask myself: Do I absolutely need it? Am I willing to take care of it? Unless I can answer yes to these questions, it stays in the store.

Along with physical decluttering, don't forget to consider how much information you want to be exposed to on a daily basis. Between newspapers, radio, TV, emails, phone calls, and the internet, we're all overloaded with information. In 2002 alone, the world produced five *quintillion* (that's 1,000,000,000,000,000,000) bytes of data—enough to fill the Library of Congress's book collection 37,000 times over!

Are you drowning in this flood? Just as you choose what objects to keep or get rid of, you can choose what information comes in and when. Instead of the disturbing news in the morning paper, I prefer solitude.

I've never even touched a computer. You can limit emails to a couple of times a day, get off email lists, decide how much time you will spend on an internet search and set a timer. Reduce your amount of TV watching and choose what you'll watch rather than leaving it on. My friend Dr. Andrew Weil even suggests eliminating the messages from TV and radio altogether. It's not about shutting out the world so much as limiting the amount and type of input. This way we have quiet to hear the soft sounds from our souls. The world screams. God whispers.

When we take time to shed useless objects and too much information, choosing what to keep and what to let go of, we get up to speed with who we are now. Let's start focusing on who we want to become. What would the ideal you think of the way you're living right now? Do you agree we have too much information and not enough self-knowledge and wisdom?

## Naomi's Clutter Busters

"I do not want my house to be walled in on all sides and my windows to be stuffed. I want the cultures of all the lands to be blown about my house as freely as possible."

—MAHATMA GANDHI

I lead a very busy life, traveling all over the country doing my weekly TV show, giving speeches, and doing publicity. In order to keep my sanity, I've developed a top eleven list for simplifying my time. It's about prioritizing my schedule! It's not about scheduling my priorities (and letting the rest slide). I try to faithfully stick to the list, which is why whenever someone comes into my home, he or she comments on how calm and peaceful it is. What's the vibe in your home? Here are some ways I make sure my haven is one letter short of heaven:

1   Start every morning with solitude to get centered and get a read on your emotional allowance.

2   Finish one thing before you go on to the next and be aware of the moment.

3   Don't stress if you don't get to everything on your list—it's never ending.

4   Answer mail and email immediately.

5   Don't keep a miscellaneous file.

6   Work somewhere with a door that can close to eliminate interruptions.

7   Buy things through catalogs and online to save time going to stores. Cancel catalogs you don't want.

8   Consolidate errands and plan your route carefully to save time.

9   Do unpleasant tasks first thing in the morning to get them over with.

10  Schedule realistically so you're not rushed and calendar in at least one day to yourself every week.

11  Learn to say no. Make promises sparingly, but keep them faithfully.

# The Missing Peace

"A man ninety years old was asked to what he attributed his longevity. 'I reckon,' he said, with a twinkle in his eye, 'it's because most nights I went to bed and slept when I should have sat up and worried.' "

—DOROTHEA KENT

It isn't just old LPs and stained blouses that we don't want to be lugging into the last phase of our lives. It's also old beliefs and emotional habits that haven't been serving us well. Have you collected too much emotional debris? Ready to do some emotional housecleaning?

Sometimes we must make these changes in order to have any kind of future. Fortunately, when I had a serious illness, mind/body/spirit experts were teaching me that stress as well as worry or fear could weaken my stressed immune system. This encouraged me to reduce as much unnecessary activity as I could in every aspect so I could have a future.

This life-saving advice is the "fountain of smart." Recent scientific research discovered long-term stress starts a civil war in our bodies that actually speeds up the aging process! It does this by changing the structure of our DNA. In a study of women under chronic stress, the most stressed women had cells that looked a whopping ten years older than their chronological age.

Stress also creates free radicals, a kind of molecule that damages DNA. We're also endangering our brains—stress hormones can shrink our hippocampus, the important part of the brain that helps in learning and remembering. This is huge! And if that doesn't motivate you to de-stress, consider this: Some scientists believe that stress in the form of anxiety or depression may increase the risk of developing Alzheimer's disease, stroke, and Parkinson's disease. Distress can be disastrous if you don't figure out a way to declutter physically, emotionally, and spiritually.

Stress is particularly dangerous for us in the twenty-first century because of the way our brains are structured. When we worry, our mind/body reacts as if we are in mortal danger. Through our nervous system, our mind/body is set up to respond to danger by setting off the fight-or-flight response: our heart rate quickens, our blood vessels constrict as our blood leaves our extremities and rushes to our core, and our bodies are flooded with adrenaline, cortisol, and other stress hormones that prepare us to fight or run. It's very effective for short-term emergencies, like being chased by a tiger in the jungle.

Unfortunately, says Robert Sapolsky, professor of biology and neuroscience at Stanford University, humans take this response designed for short-term physical emergencies and unwittingly "turn it on for months on end, worrying about mortgages, relationships, and promotions . . . or the Internal Revenue Service, about public speaking or what to say in a job interview."

And it's a vicious cycle. The more you worry, the more you flood your body with stress hormones, causing you to feel even more anxious. That's why it's so important to not be a drama queen, addicted to highly emotionally charged situations. Stress also causes us to gain weight, because in fight or flight, our bodies put out cortisol, a hormone that gives you a raging appetite which continues until the stress disappears (if it disappears!). The weight goes to our middle, as belly fat, which is associated with diabetes, some cancers, and heart disease. (Ever notice that extra weight makes someone look older than he or she is?) Inability to deal well with stress not only makes us look older and weigh more, it's literally killing us.

The opposite of worry is a sense of well-being. I want you to feel safe in the world and figure out how to handle whatever life dishes out. Once you experience that serenity, your blood vessels relax, your immune system stays strong, and the cascade of stress hormones stays switched off.

How to do it? In studies of folks who live to be a hundred, one thing that they have in common is the ability to not sweat—the small stuff, that is. These oldsters may have experienced a great deal of stress, but they choose to handle it well. For one thing, they don't take difficulties personally. They understand that an event or issue is not a personal attack on them. They've seen that people screw up a lot but are mostly doing their best. They recognize that change is inevitable so they go with the flow, even when they prefer things to be otherwise. One bad day doesn't make a bad life.

Aha! What these elders have is perspective. That's a sense of what matters in the larger scheme of things. This is the wisdom encouraged in the Serenity Prayer:

> *God grant me the serenity*
> *to accept the things I cannot change;*
> *courage to change the things I can;*
> *and wisdom to know the difference.*

## Vive la Différence!

Besides the Serenity Prayer, I destress through prayerful meditation. Scientists have found that daily meditation lowers anxiety, improves brain function, and even reduces your biological age! One study found that people who meditated for more than five years had a biological age averaging twelve years younger than nonmeditators. In another one, scientists taught meditation to a group of people in an old age home. Another group did word games. The meditators scored higher on low blood pressure, mental health—and improved ability to learn. When the researcher returned in three years, a third of the residents had died, but none were the meditators. The word *meditation* literally means "good medicine."

What also works extremely well for me in stressful times is to become aware of the preciousness of the present moment. This one right now will never come again. When I come into awareness of the immediate present, and set my focus on what is happening—the afternoon sun shining through the window, the leaves budding on the trees, the dog curled in my lap—I get centered. Worry begins to fade, because worry is always about the future, even if it's the next minute. That's what Mark Twain meant when he confessed, "I've spent most of my time worrying about things that never happened."

Present moment awareness allows me to enjoy as fully as possible what is right in front of me because I begin paying attention. My eyes, ears, and nose are engaged, my pulse and breath slow. I begin appreciating what's going on, rather than racing over it to get to the next problem or task. I call it already thereness. In a very real sense, now is all we ever have. The past is history, the future uncertain. Ever stop to notice the more we spend our time in the present moment, the more time seems to expand?

Due to the prevalence of cell phones, a new cultural phenomenon has also developed: the absent present. People are so involved in speaking on the phone, talking loudly even about intimate topics, that they are oblivious to their surroundings, whether they are in a restaurant or subway. They're not physically engaged in the present moment, and what's going on around them totally fades away. Rather than enjoying the actual experience of the moment—the sights, the sounds, the smells, the interactions—they miss out on the here and now.

I want to be alive to savor the moment. The flowers I planted outside my kitchen window. The hippy-hop of my three dogs as they race across the hardwood floor. And the more I am present, the less stress and more peace I feel emotionally, spiritually, and physically.

And for those who want to look good physically, remember: Peace of mind makes a fair face! Happiness and peace of mind can't be bought at the cosmetic counter or surgeon's office.

Sometimes, in doing our emotional truth telling, we discover that a great source of our stress is someone who's sucking our time, energy, and spirit with neediness and demands. UCLA psychiatrist Dr. Judith Orloff calls them energy vampires. Oh, yeah, you know the folks in your life I'm talking about! People who leave you feeling depleted, anxious, and depressed, rather than uplifted and energized. I'm not talking about a friend who may be going through a hard time, but those who have *only* hard times. The whiners. The naysayers or gossipers. The desperate ones who want you to save them, or at least lend an ear to endless tales of woe. They're feeding off your energy. They are not only dragging you down emotionally but taxing your immune system too.

Our time is limited. If your relationships aren't equal, in that you're both giving and receiving, you're squandering your time. The great writer Norman Cousins, who devoted the last twelve years of his life to understanding the mind/body connection, once put it this way: "Certainly we ought not to grant others the right to give us ulcers."

Sometimes we stay in relationships with energy vampires because we've known them so long that we just take their ways for granted. So now that you're aware of this information, ask yourself: If I met this person right now, would I choose to be friends? If the answer is no, for the sake of your future, how about tactfully stopping your hemorrhaging?

I stopped feeling emotionally anemic when I cut out such folks. One was someone with whom I grew up. I reached a point about fifteen years ago where I understood that she was a negative pessimist. So that's when I did the right thing for both of us. Now I just send a Christmas card once a year. The sanity you save will be your own!

## Soul Cleansing

"Life is an adventure in forgiveness."
—NORMAN COUSINS

Our souls justifiably move front and center as we're aging. In order to blossom into our ripeness, it's crucial that we clear up anything that may be obscuring our spirits. I'm now talking about that light and air for our soul—forgiveness.

Forgiveness—of ourselves and others—allows us to stay current, to shed old hurts, resentments, and toxic grudges. Only then can we put our energy on a forward-moving path. The most recent research has shown that it is good for body, mind, and soul—people who learned to forgive, particularly those over forty-five, report greater satisfaction with their lives and less nervousness, sadness, or restlessness. Coronary heart disease patients had increased blood flow to the heart after learning forgiveness. And it can even be good for your wallet—in a recent study of financial advisers, those who learned to forgive daily irritations had a 25 percent decrease in stress levels and a 25 percent increase in sales!

The reason forgiveness has positive aging benefits is that when we hold a grudge, we get stuck in the fight-or-flight response. Our brains don't know the difference between a bad memory like a grudge and a here-and-now experience. We're neither fighting nor fleeing, which traps our system in a continuous adrenalized reaction that's prematurely aging us. Conversely, forgiveness frees up our bodies to relax and our spirits to soar.

It's important to grasp that forgiveness is not about excusing the behavior that has wounded you. Nor is it necessarily about reconciling with the other person. Rather it's about coming to peace internally so that you stop carrying around the anger and hurt, furthering the damage.

Forgiveness is hard, but it's necessary for decluttering your life and growing spiritually. That's why when Jesus was asked how often he should forgive a brother who sins against him, He replied, "Seventy-seven times" (Matthew 18:22). Here are some steps I use, adapted from the Forgiveness Alliance:

1 Confront your pain—your shock, fear, anger, and grief.
   Recognize that the hurt that has occurred may have been very unfair so that these steps are not meant to minimize that hurt. You can forgive only after you have gotten in touch with and processed your fear, anger, and grief. So get the help you need—from a therapist, minister, friend—in order to do that.

2 Realize that you are the only person responsible for your own feelings. It's up to you to heal the hurt that is going on inside of you.

3 Remember that you may have had some part in what happened. Be willing to face up to that part and forgive yourself as well.

4 See this situation as motivation for healing and growth.

**5** Decide to forgive. Even if this decision is halfhearted at first, it will probably lessen your hurt and anger immediately. This decision may be difficult because you will have to give up the grudge—being the "victim," being "right" and making the other person "wrong." Notice that this is a "superior" position that can be used to get a lot of self-righteous attention. Be willing, for your sake, to have the courage to get off that "superior" position.

**6** Be willing to find a new way to think about the person who wronged you. What was his or her life like growing up? What was his or her life like at the time of the offense? What were this person's good points up to the time of the hurt? Notice that you may not be able to see much good within until you have processed out your anger and/or grief or fear.

**7** Be aware that being forgiving is a courageous act on your part. It has nothing to do with whether the other person can admit that he or she is wrong. You are forgiving to liberate yourself no matter what the other person decides to do.

**8** Turn to God for guidance and assistance in the forgiveness process.

**9** Accept the lessons involved in this incident. What have you learned from this event that is invaluable to you?

Dr. Fred Luskin's book *Forgive for Good* is my favorite on the topic because it's so practical and to the point.

# Don't Just Do Something, Sit There

"Never miss an opportunity to do nothing."
—ROGER ROSENBLATT

If you'll do the physical, emotional, and spiritual housecleaning I'm proposing, chances are you'll discover something surprising. You'll wind up with more time. Time for yourself—for rest, for solitude, for creating and enjoying the present moment. People who are stressed *out* are just that—*out*side themselves. To live from the inside out is to live by design, not chance. But to come up with an inside plan, we gotta stop and begin by doing nothing.

I reluctantly learned the benefits of inactivity when I was sick. Forced to stop moving, I gradually saw the value of rest. At first it was sooo frustrating, but now I can't imagine my day without solitude and periods of rest and alone time—time for contemplation, self-reflection. As a result, I can tell when I need to go even slower and not get caught up in the frenzy.

If we don't stop once in a while and turn our attention inward, we'll be reacting to whatever's being dished out. And we can end up, years down the line, impersonating ourselves and living a life not of our choosing.

Think you've gotten distracted from who you're meant to be? When you admit you're lost, you'll begin to find your direction. Midlife is a turning point. Like teens who must break away from their parents in order to become themselves, you and I must break away from outmoded ways of being and form new identities, roles, and lifestyles. When we spend time alone with ourselves, we have the chance, maybe for the very first time, to get in touch with who we are. In the quiet we find our deep, still center. Then our essence can begin to flow out. That way we make sure the life we lead—however many years it contains—is truly our own.

## Your Turn Now

- Are you happy to walk into your home? If not, what do you need to do so that you can be? Do you have a private space to be quiet and reflect?

- Do you need to commit to daily house decluttering? If so, visit FlyLady.net for directions and email support.

- Where are you spending your time, your most precious resource? Keep track for one week of the specific things you spend your time doing. At the end of the week, take out the list and ask yourself for each task: Does this bring me joy? Does it reduce the overall complexity of my life? If not, how can you cut it out, change it, or offload it to someone else?

- Make a to-don't list of things you don't want to do. It's a way of stopping doing too much, not guilt-tripping yourself or agonizing over things. When people request something on your list, you can simply say, "Sorry, I don't do that." End of story. My friend M.J.'s to-don'ts are ironing, making desserts, and fund-raising. Mine include handling finances and keeping track of deadlines and time lines. Life gets much simpler with a personal policy in place.

- Make a list of the top ten things that are causing you stress. Then pick one to work on getting rid of. When you've done that, go to another.

- Use these tried-and-true stress reducers: (1) Get physical. Exercise is the best stress reducer there is. Walk, run, swim, turn on the oldies and dance, hit a punching bag. I wave my arms in big circles and breathe deeply. (2) Take slow, deep breaths through the nose, making sure you fill your abdomen, not just your lungs. This stops the fight-or-flight response, assuring your body that there is no emergency. (3) Get together with (nonvampire) friends. Studies show that relationships are the best protection against stress. Positive psychologists report we're happier around others. (4) Get a massage. Among other health benefits, massage induces the relaxation response, reducing the level of stress hormones in our bodies. (5) Try saying: *Let go and let God. This too shall pass. All is well.*

- If you have habits such as perfectionism, regret, worry, problems saying no, fearfulness, negative self-talk that are cluttering your emotional closet and thereby robbing your ability to age gratefully, you should read my previous book, *Naomi's Breakthrough Guide.* You may also consider getting professional help. Lighten your load of emotional baggage so you can move ahead.

- There are many effective meditation techniques. Here's one of the best from expert Jon Kabat-Zinn and his staff at the University of Massachusetts Medical School. For years, they have been teaching meditation to patients battling chronic pain, anxiety, and depression. You may want to begin with five or ten minutes and increase the time gradually. You can do it with your eyes closed or open, depending on what's most comfortable. Sit comfortably in a chair, couch, or bed with your head, neck, and back straight but not stiff, and your shoulders relaxed. Place your hands comfortably in your lap or knees. Let your feet rest flat on the floor or stretch out. Allow your eyes slowly to close. Feel your belly gently expand and recede, rising with each in-breath and falling with each out-breath. Become aware of your feet, your legs and buttocks, and your back. Now become fully aware of your breath as it passes by your nostrils back and forth, in and out.

When thoughts arise, simply notice them and then let them go. If sensations appear in your body, notice them and let them go too. Keep bringing your attention back to your breathing each time it wanders off. Simply experience each in-breath as it comes into your body and each out-breath as it leaves your body. Feel or imagine the breath moving through your body, down into your chest, into your belly, your legs, and your toes on each in-breath and up from your toes, legs, belly, and chest on each out-breath.

As best you can, avoid judging yourself. Just note thoughts and feelings, trying not to pursue them or reject them. You see clearly what is here in this moment and then let it be. Return to your breath, maintaining moment-to-moment awareness as it continues to move in and out of your body.

■ Who depletes your energy? Who revives your energy? It's time to start telling yourself the truth. Then take action on what you feel.

- Is there someone you need to forgive? One easy way to begin is to say a forgiveness meditation out loud. Here's one by Buddhist priest Madeline Ko-I Bastis: You say the following phrase to yourself: *For all the harm you have done me, knowingly or unknowingly, I forgive you as much as I can.* If it's yourself you need to forgive, change the words accordingly. Say it a few times a day until you don't need to anymore. If you feel resistance when you say it, try this: *I am willing to forgive, but not yet.*

- Do you take time for yourself every day? How comfortable are you in solitude? Can you carve out at least twenty minutes for yourself in which you do absolutely nothing? For example, I try to lie flat for a half hour every afternoon when I am home.

- How often are you able to be purposefully in the present? Do you spend most of your time in the future, worrying over what might be? Or in the past, shoulding all over yourself? When you catch yourself there, come back to the present moment by engaging your senses. What can you see? What can you hear? What does it feel like to sit on the chair?

# 4 | *Good Will Hunting:* Finding Purpose and Meaning

I NEVER SET OUT to be a celebrity of any kind. Or a singer. Or a writer. As a single mom, I wanted to make enough money for rent, food, and clothing, and to take care of Wy and Ashley. I found my work as a nurse fulfilling, but I was away from home too much. Every day I was consumed with getting a paycheck in order to get the kids shoes. Purpose back then meant making ends meet and keeping my kids safe.

But as Wy grew into her teenage years, I could see that she had phenomenal musical ability. Sending a young girl out into the wild world of country music alone was unthinkable. So I began to sing harmony. I wanted to enhance her efforts and let her become who she was meant to be. In a way, the Judds were born to give her life meaning. My motherly purpose was to protect and encourage.

There are no words to describe how much I loved being with Wy and singing. But the serendipitous connections we made with all the different people on the road as we toured in the bus also gave me great satisfaction—much greater satisfaction than the recording contracts, the awards, and the fame. I depended on the way music connected us to one another as well as to other human beings. We were soon sharing stories with many different personalities from diverse backgrounds.

Over time, it became apparent that my sense of fulfillment came from tapping into what I consider my soul's purpose. The closest I can come to naming my purpose is to say that it's about healing myself and then offering what works to help others. And when I share what I've figured out—in an interview, a TV show, or the books I've written—that offers reinforcement of ideas and gives further insights. The process of helping others is a form of prayer, because it aligns me with what brings me closer to God. It connects me to my own innate divinity. Whatever gifts God's given me are my talents. I show my gratitude by using them to honor Him. Have you found your soul's purpose? Can you name it?

After I was diagnosed with hepatitis C and spent an intense time being sick and depressed, the feeling of wanting to help others never wavered. Waiting to have blood drawn in hospital labs, I'd try to comfort other patients. To add insult to injury, I was forced to retire in my late forties. I lost my livelihood and my career. It was a crossroads. What's left? I wondered. Doctors said I had no future, but I wasn't afraid of dying. I was worried about finding a different way to live my purpose.

Alone, I lay in bed or sat at my kitchen table, day after day, week after week, staring out into my valley, and struggled. What shall I do with myself? Previously, I slept on a bus with Wy and woke up in a new town every day. One day, Madison Avenue in New York; then San Antonio, Texas, the next. I'd open the bus curtains and be exposed to experiences no one could predict. Every night we were surrounded by thousands of people. Now Larry confronted me for not even brushing my hair for days on end or getting out of my PJs. He insisted I had to initiate a change. My doctor prescribed an antidepressant.

I chose to have a breakthrough instead of a breakdown. I chose to have a new growth experience based on an idea for a new purpose. In order to find my purpose, I needed to consider what my gifts and inclinations were, what my disposition is, and what I'd learned through my circumstances.

You might use my discovery as an example. I knew I had some raw talent as a storyteller and I love people. I'd just finished my autobiography, and writing it had afforded me awareness by stepping back and looking objectively at what had happened in my life so far. That experience finally taught me that my purpose is to walk the path of healer and teacher. I found meaning in my connection with fans, with what I'd learned in my medical research about hep C, the cutting-edge scientific research into the mind/body/spirit connection, and human behavior as a nurse. What if I took all this and spoke about it? Wrote about it? And so I pulled myself up by my bootstraps and took a risk. I contacted a speakers' bureau and my new career as lecturer and author was born. Evolutionary scientist Charles Darwin said, "It's not the smartest or the strongest of a species that survives. It's the ones that are willing to adapt." As I discovered, aging gratefully requires being flexible and adaptable to ever-changing circumstances.

## *Set Your Feet on a Path That's Going Somewhere*

"Life's one imperative is to become who we are."
—THOMAS MERTON

Let's stop and look back at how we've gotten this far. I got the idea to become a nurse to fulfill my need to help lessen suffering. Then my purpose shifted to guiding Wy into a career in country music. Our adventures as the Judds allowed me to multiply the number of people I could reach out to. I was exposed to unbelievable opportunities to help others in new ways. I took full advantage of this myriad of avenues for learning. Through it all, in spite of mistakes, I have been intentionally living my purpose.

Question: Do you feel like the first part of your life essentially has been a mistake? Were you so busy learning how to please parents, fit in at school, find a lover, earn a living, be a parent, etc., that you're just now able to become that individual you know you are meant to be?

You may not have had any control over beliefs imprinted on you by early memories and experiences. Additionally, the superficial, youth-oriented society all around you probably had a detrimental influence.

James Hollis, a Jungian analyst and author of *Finding Meaning in the Second Half of Life: How to Finally, Really Grow Up*, believes that however productive or well-meaning our first decades were, midlife is the important crossroads where we choose our destiny. I agree. I was thirty-eight when we signed with RCA.

Did your beliefs, the way you grew up, and the way you tried to conform keep your inner longings from developing? Now you can find your values—what you feel in your bones, whatever matters most. How would others describe you? I've been called eccentric, a colorful character, and an idealist. You no longer need anybody's permission to say and do exactly what you're feeling. Andy Rooney on *60 Minutes* said, "Older women can be so dignified. They won't throw a drink in your face at a restaurant or cause a scene in public. They might just shoot you, though."

Will the real you stand up? Don't be timid—it's the decision you're supposed to be making at this stage. Your future is like an idea in your womb: as you consider your needs, you form new parts. Restless, unsatisfied? Starting to feel pangs? You'll eventually rebirth your authentic self. I'm your coach gently urging, "Take a deep breath. Push, push." Your purpose here on planet Earth is to discover your purpose.

Spiritual leader Marianne Williamson believes, "Every change is a challenge to become who we really are." No matter what our life circumstances have been, no matter what crossroads we now find ourselves at—empty nest, retirement, divorce, burnout, feeling blah—we are supposed to take everything we've learned and bring it to bear on determining the rest of our life.

Purpose is a sense that your life has some larger dimension to it, some quest that you must pursue. It has no specific end. It's the emotion at the center of our being. It may seem ordinary to others, but it has a sense of holiness to us. My friend, best-selling author Caroline Myss, writes about how our lives aren't random events but a charted course of opportunities. Not guarantees, but opportunities.

Purpose is different from goals. To learn to fly a small plane, as one sixty-five-year-old acquaintance just did, is a goal. To empower the youth of tomorrow by teaching adults to read is purpose.

The idea of who you can be is just beginning. When life expectancy was only forty-seven, survival was our grandparents' dominating purpose. They didn't get the benefit of this second chance. The generation of baby boomers are illustrating that the sky's not the limit. Speaking of which . . . baby boomer Sally Ride was the first woman in space.

Winston Churchill is considered one of the great figures of the twentieth century. When he was elected British prime minister at age sixty-four, he reflected, "All my life has been spent preparing to be prime minister." This realization should be true for us all. Everything that has happened to us—the good and the bad—has helped weave a pattern of purpose in our lives. That's why it's also important to look for clues in the hardships we've lived through, as well as what we love and are good at.

In January 2006, sixty-seven-year-old Ellen Johnson-Sirleaf was named the first female president of the war-torn African country of Liberia. Liberians say she's the "best chance for peace they have ever known." Nicknamed "The Iron Lady," she's committed to using everything she learned about injustice. Liberia will no longer use children as soldiers.

At the same time, Chile named a new president—Michelle Bachelet, a fifty-four-year-old pediatrician and single mom. Bachelet had been imprisoned and tortured under the dictatorship of General Pinochet.

When we are knee-deep in our fear and difficulties, it can be hard to realize at the time that such challenges bring out our strengths as well as spotlight our weaknesses. I'm encouraging you to look at them that way. Whatever your current hardship is, consider it as a test to define you. In this way, all our difficulties have meaning.

Consider the case of Candy Lightner, who started Mothers Against Drunk Driving after her thirteen-year-old daughter was killed by a drunk driver. Or Doris Tate, the mother of Sharon Tate, the actress who was murdered by the Manson family in 1969. Doris sank into depression after her daughter's death but emerged to become a victims' rights advocate. She was the first member of a victim's family ever to speak at a parole hearing and campaigned to make such statements law. Such a law has now been adopted throughout the country.

These women found their calling through unspeakable tragedy, and I certainly hope you will never have to face anything so terrible. But no life is without its difficulties. Can you begin to look for what your challenges are trying to tell you? Then grit your teeth and see if you're contributing to a bad situation. Don't repeat what's bad—keep and repeat the good lessons.

Finding meaning in adversity is also good for our health. Researchers discovered that it helps lower stress hormone levels in breast cancer patients, leads to fewer recurring heart attacks in cardiac patients, and improves immune functioning and lowers mortality among those who suffered the death of a loved one. Finding meaning has also been found to aid emotional adjustment and lessen depression after a loss of a family member and after combat exposure. When I realized there's no public awareness of hep C, which will kill four times more Americans than AIDS this decade, I was so distressed that I formed the Naomi Judd Research and Education Fund for Hepatitis C. Every time I speak about this killer, I'm feeling better and fulfilling a purpose.

The poet William Wordsworth put it this way: "A deep distress hath humanized my soul." Our body, mind, and spirit are balanced when we discover a higher purpose. However, you don't have to go through difficulties to experience the benefits of purpose and meaning. UCLA scientists have discovered that *whenever* we find meaning in our lives, we get a boost in our immune function.

Many great movies, like *Star Wars,* are based on seeing your life as a mythic journey. The hero—that's you—sets out on some kind of quest and faces all kinds of challenges. These challenges make him or her stronger, better, more kind and wise. And he or she then finds a purpose and goes on to help others. You can go from victim to hero too.

When we contemplate our lives in this metaphorical way, we understand that purpose is what casts us as heroes of our own story. As we age, what's going on in our face is so much less important that what's going on in our heart and head. When times are tough for me, rather than getting stuck in self-pity or blame, I ask myself: What is this situation trying to teach me? What else can I learn about myself? How can I offer what I'm learning to encourage or inspire someone else in this predicament?

Viktor Frankl, who survived the Holocaust, believed: "There is nothing in this world, I venture to say, that would so effectively help one survive even the worst conditions as the knowledge there is meaning in one's life."

## Go with the Flow

"Perhaps the greatest boost to self-confidence is the embrace of a larger-than-self purpose. Instead of worrying about how we are being perceived or judged by others, we can devote ourselves to important work. . . . Self-confidence is nothing special. It is the absence of self-consciousness, nothing more, nothing less."
—LAURENCE BOLDT

When was the last time you were in such a happy state of mind, experiencing such complete engagement, that you got lost in an activity? When Wy and I were recording in the studio, we lost track of time. Only our stomachs growling made us stop and eat. Ashley completely loses herself in her movie roles. Mihaly Csikszentmihalyi, professor of social science at the Peter Drucker School of Business at Claremont University, taught me about this state of mind he calls flow. When we're involved fully in a task, we can enjoy it so thoroughly that time and self-awareness disappear. Csikszentmihalyi has found that feeling of flow is most likely to occur when we are neither bored nor anxious but are using our strengths on behalf of something really challenging that matters to us. When Grace, my granddaughter, is baking cookies with me, or Elijah, my grandson, is skateboarding, they are in the flow. What task are you doing when this flow happens for you?

Csikszentmihalyi and his colleagues have collected millions of samples of flow by randomly beeping their subjects throughout the day and finding out how engaged they are. They've discovered that those who experience flow are happier than others. Those who don't experience flow tend not to challenge themselves in any way—they hang out at malls more, watch more TV. They have more leisure time but don't know what to do with it; they often feel bored and unhappy. They may think they want *more* leisure, but what they really are craving is more meaningful and challenging activity.

What Csikszentmihalyi and other social scientists have discovered is that while too much stress is bad for you, not enough stimulation is harmful too. For instance, folks who sleep more than nine hours a night tend to die younger. And a large percentage of people die within three years of retirement. Our mind/body/spirit systems are meant to experience the 4 Cs: to meet challenges, to exert control, to make commitments to things that matter to us, and to stay connected to life and to other people.

When we live with the 4 Cs, our life force remains strong. If we don't, our systems respond by shutting down: Party's over? I'm outta here. Part of the art of aging, then, is to find ways and places to practice the 4 Cs. Don't expect them to track us down in front of our TV. We must go out of ourselves and our houses to experience flow and purpose.

Flow is such a desired state that Walter M. Bortz II, past president of the American Geriatric Society, says, "He or she who dies with the most flow is a success." Here's another benefit to aging gratefully: The experience of flow is something that can increase with age *if* we pay attention. As Bortz says, "Our repertoire of talents is greater" than younger people's. And our "ability to distinguish what matters from what doesn't is greater, so that focus is greater." We're "less self-conscious, and since self-consciousness is incompatible with flow, [we] have another advantage. I can't wait to grow older so I can have more flow."

Me too! The more we live out our purpose, the more we will experience being in the flow. We're rewarded with feelings of usefulness and bliss.

## Following Your Bliss, No Matter Your Age

"It's never too late to be what you might have been."
—GEORGE ELIOT

What I've discovered in my own life—and psychologists agree it's generally true—is that the desire to be in touch with our purpose grows stronger as we age. When we're young, we get excited by fame or fortune, by all the material goodies the media tries to tantalize us with. But as we grow older, we figure out firsthand that this stuff doesn't deliver contentment. The whispers of our soul grow louder until we can no longer ignore them.

When Ashley was a teen in college in the U.K., she volunteered at a soup kitchen once a week. She's always had a purposeful activity. As a famous leading lady in major films, she's around the glitz and glamour trappings of Hollywood. Sweetpea loves her career and considers portraying diverse human behaviors enlightening. But in her personal quest for purpose and meaning she's also a global ambassador for Youth AIDS. As I pen these words, she's in the slums of Africa teaching sex workers to protect themselves with condoms and promoting abstinence and birth control. I can't imagine what Ashley'll be like as she ages!

The great thinker Joseph Campbell put it this way: "You may have success in life, but then ask yourself—what kind of life was it? What good was it if you've never done the thing you wanted to do all your life or went where your heart and soul wanted to go? When you find that feeling, stay with it, and don't let anyone throw you off."

## Pull the Ripcord and Jump

"It takes courage to grow up and turn out to be who you really are."
—E. E. CUMMINGS

Sherry Lansing is one smart cookie and she doesn't crumble. I met her when she was the first female head of Paramount Studios. She's a perfect example of realizing when it's time to reinvent yourself. Stepping down from her job, Sherry confided, "I loved my job the whole time . . . but . . . I didn't want to die at my desk without having explored whatever else might be out there. . . . I think, at sixty, it's time. At sixty, finally, you've earned the right to be authentic."

Being authentic means behaving in accordance with your values and doing what you believe, regardless of what someone else tells you. It's refusing to settle for less and doing what you know is right.

To become authentic can be challenging at any age. It takes courage. The word *courage* comes from the Latin *cor*, meaning "heart." When we are "at heart," we can face the demons of self-doubt that stand between us and what we truly want. Don't you think I was scared when I first stood on an empty stage without Wy and our band to give my first speech? Or the first time I interviewed someone for my TV show? Of course. But the prospect of helping others in ways that mattered deeply to me gave me courage. I recalled all the other first times I'd made it through.

Life purpose coach Richard Leider in his book *Claiming Your Place at the Fire* asks: "What would you be doing if you were ten times more courageous in the second half of your life than you were in the first?" How will *you* answer that question? What we need is nothing less than the courage to be ourselves.

For many of us, one of the biggest concerns at this time in our lives is that it's too late, we're too old, we've missed our chance. Phooey! Age is no obstacle to creativity or success when we've decided to set our feet on our soul's path. Every awareness we have of our age is our soul actually confirming the importance of making good use of the time remaining.

My friend Paul McLemore, who's fifty-one, married, and responsible for three kids at home, recently summoned up his courage to become his authentic self. All his adult life Paul's been traveling during weekdays selling heavy machinery. Tired of staying in Hampton Inns and being away from his growing family, he yearned to try his hand at selling land and being home for supper at his table. Giving up his medical insurance and 401(k) was terrifying. His nervous wife, Suzanne, told me I may see her at the grocery store asking "paper or plastic?" until he gets a sale, but now they're the happiest they've ever been.

The authors of the New England Centenarian Study share stories of folks over a hundred who found meaning at the century mark through following their dreams and passions—the Senior Olympics competitor, the bridge champion, the poet. These folks are proof that it's never too late to find or reclaim untapped or unexplored aspects of ourselves.

One of my favorite centenarians is Anna Morgan, who, at age one hundred, despite "cataracts, glaucoma, and macular degeneration . . . read a newspaper each day . . . placed telephone calls and stuffed envelopes for local groups, such as Mobilization for Survival. During her nineties, she wrote more than 1,200 pages of memoirs, a portion of which were published. . . . She also worked on an effort for a postal stamp to commemorate the black singer, actor, and political figure Paul Robeson." Anna Morgan was not unique—each of the centenarians, researchers found, had a full day's activities each and every day. As 103-year-old sculptor Beatrice Woods told reporters, "It's only the covering that grows old."

Here are a few other examples for inspiration. Colonel Harland Sanders started Kentucky Fried Chicken at age sixty-five—and sold it at seventy-four. Frank Lloyd Wright designed the Guggenheim Museum at age ninety. Benjamin Franklin invented bifocals at seventy-eight (he probably needed them by then!). Grandma Moses *painted* at one hundred. The composer Leopold Stokowski signed a six-year recording contract at ninety-four. Monet began painting his water lilies at seventy-six. Barbara McClintock won the Nobel Prize in medicine at age eighty-one. In the study on aging done on nuns, researcher David Snowdon describes lively Sister Esther. She was a teacher—at ninety-two, having gotten her master's in theology at age seventy-one. "I'm too busy to be in a study of old people," she told Snowdon. None of these folks allowed the age on the page to interfere with the person they wanted to become. They just followed their purpose and passion. I say, people who don't ever get carried away ought to try it!

I've found it a relief that aging allows us to follow our passions without the pressure of recognition or reward. Released from having to prove something or make a living at something, we can more freely just be ourselves. I was so self-conscious when the Judds began. When I watch old videos, I squirm when I see how obviously hard I was trying.

We're free to break stereotypes too. Lowell Tozer, seventy-six, is one of only three men volunteers in a hospital cuddler's program, in which he holds and rocks premature babies. He's always loved babies, but this was his first volunteer job. "Had I known I could be doing this in retirement, I would have retired sooner," he exclaims. He loves it so much that he talked the hospital into letting him come three days a week, rather than the standard three hours a week.

No one exemplifies finding and struggling to live your purpose fully more than Oprah. Now in her fifties, she says, "How do I accelerate my humanity? How do I use who I am on earth for a purpose that's bigger than myself? How do I align the energy of my soul with my personality . . . to serve my soul? My answer always comes back to self. There is no moving up and out into the world unless you are fully acquainted with who you are. You cannot move freely, speak freely, act freely, and be free unless you are comfortable with yourself." She added, "All these years I've been feeling . . . like I was growing into myself. Finally, I feel grown."

Sometimes the path of purpose is not a straight line. At age thirty-eight I was signed, along with Wy, to a record contract with RCA. Wy was the youngest person ever signed (besides Elvis) and I was the oldest. Until then, I had not had any medical coverage, any kind of insurance, or a savings account. During our eight years as the Judds, we were undefeated at every award show. At age sixty in 2006, I was named one of the humanitarians of the year and awarded the AARP Impact Award for my activism against poverty. Co-awardee Michael J. Fox was acknowledged for his work fighting Parkinson's disease and for advocating for stem cell research. Michael and I agreed we both miss our entertainment lives. But we also concurred that the work we're committed to now is exactly what we're supposed to be doing. (I put my Impact Award beside my Grammys.)

Sitting on my studio set in New York for my Hallmark Channel show *Naomi's New Morning,* it dawned on me that I am now communicating my beliefs and values on a huge scale. And I'm facilitating others as they fulfill their purpose! The guests are extremely passionate and expert in valuable subjects, like my own life coach Ted Klontz, PhD, an expert on family issues. Experts like Joan Borysenko, PhD, and Candace Pert, PhD, both instrumental in my healing, got to tell the world about their research on how what we're thinking can increase or decrease immune function. And regular folks like a guy who trains dogs to detect cancer or a woman who teaches dogs to alert their owners before a seizure occurs so they can prepare. Every week I am privileged to meet new people with new ideas. Sometimes we need to let go of the life we had to begin the one we're supposed to have.

## *Your Turn Now*

- What was your first thought as a child of what you'd be when you grew up? Does that still have a pull for you now?

- What is left for you to learn in your life? To give to others? Journal for ten minutes your answers to these questions. Then do it again, using the hand you don't normally write with (don't worry that it's messy). You'll be hearing from your untrained mind, so what comes up may be surprising.

- What are your unique talents? If you're not sure, you can go to www.ptp-partners.com and order their thinking talent cards. It has helped me a lot to understand mine. Our talents are the raw materials that we use to create our purpose.

- Consider volunteering for an organization to get your feet wet and see if it spurs your further interest. Older citizens are usually more concerned about and informed on political issues. Volunteer at your party headquarters.

- Write a sentence that describes your purpose. It doesn't have to be fancy. Remember mine? Healing myself and others. One way to think about it is to ask yourself where you have been willing to take a stand in your life. Or what cause you feel passionate about. Ask yourself: If I could teach something, what would I teach? Whom would I teach it to? When you say or read it, if you get a yes in your body, you've got it.

- Another way to get at purpose is to imagine yourself at the end of your life. Imagine that your whole life is like a thread. You will be asked one question that will serve as a needle that will thread your life. What is the question you want to be asked? Here are some other people's responses: Have you loved yourself? Have you made a difference? Have you been as big as you could have been in the world? Use your question as your purpose guide, checking in with it frequently.

- Do you remember your dreams? Dreams can help us reconnect with the abandoned parts of ourselves and reclaim them. Begin keeping a dream journal and see what messages your deeper self has to give you.

- According to the Indian health system called Ayurveda, a person's life is supposed to span a hundred years, divided into four twenty-five-year parts. The first twenty-five years is about learning about life and yourself, the second is for raising a family, the third is about offering your talents to the larger community, and the last is for reflection and developing greater connection to God. Where are you in the cycle? What were the major events of each stage? What have you learned in each stage about your purpose?

- Is there a dream or passion that you had to sacrifice because you had children to raise? A career you've always wanted to try? Imagine there was nothing holding you back, what would you want to do? If you were to die right now, what would you regret not having done? It's never too late to reclaim those aspects of yourself that were left by the wayside.

- If you had all the money you needed, what would you want to do with yourself? How can you do more of that anyway?

- Want to find work? Try the following websites that cater to midlife folks and beyond: www.retiredbrains.com, www.senioriobbank.org, www.civicventures.org, www.thephoennixlink.com.

- To find out more about Youth AIDS, a global initiative that fights the spread of AIDS/HIV among the world's youth that Ashley is the spokesperson for, go to www.youthaids.org.

"To keep the heart unwrinkled, to be hopeful, kindly, cheerful . . .
that is to triumph over old age."

—THOMAS BAILEY ALDRICH

# 5 | *Where the Heart Is:* Practicing Positivism, Gratitude, and Generosity

THREE IMPORTANT WORDS describe how I've survived all obstacles so far—positivism, gratitude, and generosity. They are in part why I continue to thrive, and how you can join me in aging gratefully.

In a very literal way, being positive was as important as medicine in facilitating my cure from hep C. Doctors predicted that, with the way my liver disease was escalating, I had only three years to live. Imagine for a second you've just had a liver biopsy and some medical experts have convened to present their prognosis. Factor in that you feel like crap and have felt that way for a year. Would you accept such an authoritative opinion? I'm still alive and kicking because I didn't. A pessimist probably would have bought into their medical curse, like a voodoo hex. I snapped when I heard that prognosis. I got mad. Yeah, even furious. How many more impressionable patients, I wondered, had they sent to a six-foot dirt nap via the power of suggestion?

Something happened in my gut when I heard that death sentence. I sensed that our human body moves along the path of our expectations, whatever they are. Your beliefs become your biology. I believed it wasn't my time to die. I began asking questions and researching how positive beliefs could help my body. What I later learned from experts is how powerfully our thoughts affect our health.

If I allowed myself to be pessimistic, my stress hormones might have impaired my immune system and the virus would have gone rampant. So instead, I flipped a mental switch when I felt doubt and fear. I just decided to feel better. Optimism is good physical medicine. It not only stops the cascade of harmful stress biochemicals, it encourages fighter cells. I started "thinking positive" and that—along with other enlightening physical, mental, and spiritual practices, and finally finding Dr. Right—allowed me to recover fully.

Now, even though I am radiantly healthy, I make an effort to practice optimism every day. When something is not going the way I want it to, I remember the mind/body connection. I saw how positivism benefited my own life and I now have collected reams of medical evidence to support it. I've had so much pain in my life that now I really want to enjoy every drop of every day. As I work with hep C sufferers, I ask them to name illnesses that were deadly in the early 1900s. Typhoid fever, diphtheria, polio. I point out that these fatal diseases are no longer a danger because of vaccines or cures. I encourage them to stay positive because I believe we'll likewise soon find cures for viruses like hep C, cancer, etc. (If someone you know is suffering from hep C, please check out my website at www.NaomiJudd.com and give him or her this book!) You can also get information from the American Liver Foundation or check for a hep C support group in your area.

# Happiness Has No Expiration Date

"No matter how old you are, there's always something good to look forward to."

—LYNN JOHNSTON

So, as I discovered in my late forties in the midst of a life-threatening illness, it's never too late to start being happy. I remembered patients I cared for who were seriously ill but still found some small activity or object to make them smile. They healed much sooner. No matter our age, health status, or physical appearance, one of the best things we can do for ourselves is to stay focused on the positive. Why is this so important? It turns out that our brains actually reward us for our good thoughts with better all-around health. This allows us to live longer.

As a patient, I was frustrated that modern medicine focuses only on disease and dying. Likewise, mental health used to be concerned only with depression, anxiety, phobias, etc. Both sciences were half-baked. Mental health advocates now recognize that mental health is much more than the absence of illness. Hence, positive psychology now studies what makes people happy and well. Here's how the brain works. The thinking part of our brain is called the neocortex. Its two lobes, the left and the right, do different activities. In the past ten years, breakthroughs in technology such as magnetic resonance imaging (MRI), which measures blood flow; electroencephalograms (EEGs), which measure electrical activity; and PET (position-emission tomography) scans showing the brain's activity have allowed researchers to "see" positive thinking. As a result, we now know more about the functioning of our brains than ever before.

One of the most amazing things scientists have discovered is that the brain is like a drugstore. When we think positive thoughts—hopefulness, thankfulness, optimism, kindness—we use our left prefrontal cortex and flood our bodies with endorphins, the body's natural feel-good chemicals. Endorphins are also the body's painkillers. They help lower blood pressure by dilating blood vessels and slowing heart rate.

When you concentrate on positive thoughts, these positive chemical showers translate into major health benefits for healthy aging. For instance, people who score high in happiness tests create 50 percent more antibodies in response to a flu vaccine than the average person. A positive outlook has been shown to reduce pain in cancer patients. Got your attention now? And several studies have reported recently that optimistic older people are less likely to develop Alzheimer's disease, develop colds, or die prematurely, and they have a reduced risk for heart disease, diabetes, and high blood pressure.

They take better care of themselves too! In a forty-year study of two hundred Harvard undergraduates, having a positive attitude at twenty-five was a predictor of good health at sixty-five. Those who were highly pessimistic at twenty-five tended to be dead by the age of sixty-five. A study that followed folks between the ages of sixty-five and eighty-five found that optimists had a 55 percent lower risk of death.

I am so excited about this research, which surprised even scientists. Here's another amazing one: Harvard professor Laura Kubzansky found that over ten years, optimists were 50 percent less likely to have a heart attack than pessimists, as big a difference as between nonsmokers and smokers! Dr. Kubzansky said in a *Time* magazine article, "I'm an optimist, but I didn't expect results like this."

I love the passage in Proverbs that expresses the power of positivism that science is now discovering: "A merry heart does good like a medicine, but a broken spirit drieth the bones." One of the most fascinating studies that prove this point comes from Dr. David Snowdon, who, for almost twenty years, has been studying a group of 678 Catholic nuns, ages 75–106, who kept diaries when they entered the convent in their youth. When the diaries were analyzed for upbeat thoughts, they discovered that positive emotions added on average 6.9 years to a nun's life expectancy.

But what's happening when we think negatively? When we are worried, fearful, angry, depressed, or pessimistic, we activate our right prefrontal cortex and flood our bodies with harmful stress hormones such as cortisol and adrenaline. Uh-oh. These constrict blood vessels, raising our blood pressure and potentially damaging arteries and the heart, which increases the risk of stroke and heart attack. Stroke is the number three killer of Americans, 160,000 people every year. Our immune system weakens as the production of natural killer cells goes down. That's why people who tend to the gloomy side die earlier— they've been stressing their systems for decades. They literally put themselves out of their own misery.

I've been focusing on physical benefits, but choosing to think on the bright side has social and emotional benefits as well. Who would you rather be around? Someone grousing and complaining all the time, or a cheerful person who has a ready smile and an upbeat word to say? Folks who are optimistic naturally attract people to them like bees to pollen and therefore tend to have a more active social life. And because they are then flooding their bodies with feel-good hormones all the time, they get to feel good emotionally as well. They have more energy and look eagerly forward to the future, because they expect more good things will happen. Scientists have found that optimism is one of the key predictors of happiness, no matter our age or income.

Optimism also helps create success. Because when you expect

good things to happen, you help manifest them. I know that's been true for me. Once, while performing at a rodeo, I heard a story about a bull rider. For the first six months of riding, he focused on all that could go wrong: "Oh, no, what if I get thrown before eight seconds?" (To be a bull rider, you must stay on the bull for eight seconds.) "What if I get trampled by the bull? What if I get paralyzed? What if I get killed?" He kept falling off and losing. After the first six months, he reconsidered: "Wait a minute. Let me think about this differently. What if I focus my mental energy instead on what could go right and how I'll deal with that? What will I do with all the money I make? What will I do about all the fans after me?" And he started to win. He is now the United States bull-riding champion.

What scientists are now discovering is that each of us has a "tilt"— a tendency for either our left or right prefrontal lobe to get activated no matter what is happening. In other words, as we go about our day, some of us are feeling great, because we're thinking positive thoughts and our left prefrontal lobe is producing the feel-good chemicals. Others, even in similar circumstances, are thinking negative thoughts and activating the right side. Not only are they feeling stressed and anxious, but they're also opening their bodies up to disease.

About 50 percent of the satisfaction we feel about our lives is programmed by our genetics. We all have a certain happiness set point— whatever our external circumstances, we tend to gravitate back to the same general happiness level. In other words, we may tilt to the left or the right no matter what is going on. However, as researchers and the rodeo rider found out, if we have a tendency to go to the gloomy right, we can train ourselves to tilt toward the left, becoming more positive and therefore healthier and happier. That's where our ability to choose our attitude and influence our health and happiness comes in! Optimism is trainable, like riding a bike. Or a bull.

# Give Your 'Tude Some Altitude

"It is essential to learn to enjoy life. It really does not make sense to go through the motions of existence if one does not appreciate as much of it as possible."

—MIHALY CSIKSZENTMIHALYI

The main expert in the field of positive emotions is Martin Seligman, who years ago pioneered the study of the differences between optimistic and pessimistic thinking. His goal is to help those of us who don't naturally focus on the positive. He shows us how to choose "learned optimism."

Optimistic thinkers tend to see negative events as merely temporary conditions that are related to specific events outside their control. My husband snapped at me today because of work frustrations, not because of something wrong in our marriage. I saw it as a temporary thing that wasn't my fault and knew that he would feel better in an hour. It's really not about me.

Pessimistic folks, on the other hand, tend to see negative events as permanent, pervasive, and their fault: I am a terrible wife, he has always hated me, it's my fault for not being perfect.

When it comes to positive events, however, the situation is reversed: Optimists see good things as the result of permanent, lasting qualities of themselves (I got a bonus because I'm smart) while pessimists view them as temporary, chance events outside of their control (I won because for once, I got lucky). Because they believe good outcomes are within their control and the bad things are flukes, optimists tend to work harder next time to achieve their goal. Conversely, pessimists tend to blame themselves and give up—it went wrong because I can't succeed at anything; what's the use of even trying?

To go from pessimism to optimism, says Seligman, you must change the way you explain the good and bad things that happen to you. Become aware of your internal dialogue. When things go right in your life, you should ask yourself: What about me made this wonderful thing happen? And when things go wrong, remind yourself: This particular situation is temporary. It is confined to this one time or thing. It is outside of my control.

When I talk about choosing optimism, I use the word *practice*. That's because that's what it takes—practicing over and over. That's what learned optimism needs—a continuous commitment to be aware of your mental energy every day, until it becomes such a habit that it gets automatic.

The good news is that it *does* get easier. The more you think in a positive fashion, the more you strengthen the pathways in your brain to that way of thinking. Old brains can learn new tricks—but it takes motivation and practice (three weeks, say some researchers).

You'll be doing your blood pressure a favor too. A study of a hundred middle-age folks found that optimists scored about five points lower than pessimists on blood pressure readings.

# Healthy, Happy Heart

"The invariable mark of wisdom is to see the miraculous in the common."

—RALPH WALDO EMERSON

I've started calling gratitude vitamin G because of all the beneficial effects we're learning about it. There's a reason why I called this book

*Aging Gratefully.* The more you can value and appreciate whatever you have, the happier and more fulfilled the rest of your days will be.

Gratitude is a sense, as Benedictine monk David Steindl-Rast says, that makes our hearts feel a "great fullness." When I think thoughts of appreciation, I fill up empty spaces in myself. Life feels worth living. Grateful thoughts, like optimistic ones, activate our left prefrontal cortex and flood our bodies with those desirable endorphins.

When I studied the power of gratitude, I uncovered all kinds of positive mental, emotional, and physical effects. For instance, folks who wrote down their blessings just once a week were significantly more satisfied than those who did not.

And listen to this one! People who wrote down every day what they were thankful for not only had a big jump in happiness and energy but also took better care of themselves. See, gratitude does help us live longer. They exercised more regularly, got checkups, and wore their seat belts and sunscreen. It turns out that when you are thankful, you recognize your health as a gift and therefore care for it better. (By the way, another group in the study had to write down every hassle and problem in their day. They were the most unhappy and least healthy, so if you keep a journal, make sure you are recording all the wonderful things in your life, not the gloomy ones.) To acknowledge the anniversary of my birth, each year I make appointments for all my doctor checkups—eyes checked, teeth cleaned, mammogram, Pap smear, etc. I celebrate my health and take responsibility for keeping tabs.

People who are grateful are less attached to material possessions, less likely to be envious of others, and more willing to share. Gratefulness also helps you move toward goals, both interpersonal and health-based, have more positive energy, have better relationships and work life, feel a greater connection to others and to God, experience less depression, anger, and stress, even sleep better!

Maybe you're asking, "But what about all the terrible happenings in the world? What about all the hardships in my life?" Expressing gratitude is not about denying difficulties. It's healthy to grieve, say no, set limits, even to get appropriately angry. But it's not either/or. Being grateful is about paying attention to whatever is right at any moment even though not *everything* is right. Psychologist Robert Emmons explains it this way: "To say we feel grateful is not to say that everything is necessarily great. It just means we are aware of our blessings." Remember, someone else may be responsible for the circumstance, but you are responsible for your reactions to them. Hey, that's something to be grateful for!

My good friend Mary Jane Ryan wrote the popular book *Attitudes of Gratitude.* She tells a personal story: "I went to see my father in the hospital about a week before he died. He had suffered for years with emphysema, hooked up to an oxygen tank, barely able to move around, and was failing fast. Bedridden, he was on constant oxygen and medication, his six-foot-two frame weighed only 130 pounds because eating anything but ice cream was too difficult. Every breath was a labored struggle. I asked him whether the quality of his life was worth all the effort. 'I still enjoy being alive,' he responded. 'Sometimes it's easier to breathe and then I really enjoy just quietly taking a breath. I still enjoy reading the comics in the newspaper and watching the ball games on TV. My life is good.' " In the midst of all his terrible difficulties, M.J.'s father was able to focus on the few things that were still right, and as a consequence, enjoyed himself as much as possible to the end.

Some people don't take advantage of this built-in upper because they confuse thoughts and feelings. They mistakenly think we must wait around until we *feel* grateful in order to experience it. But it's the other way around. Good feelings *follow* thoughts. So think about what's positive and right, and you soon will feel better. It will become a habit.

# Bring More Gratitude into Your Everyday Moments

"Gratitude unlocks the fullness of life. It turns what we have into enough, and more. It turns denial into acceptance, chaos into order, confusion to clarity. . . . Gratitude makes sense of our past, brings peace for today, and creates a vision for tomorrow."

—MELODY BEATTIE

Ever talk to a person who has had a near-death experience? Most folks to whom this has happend lose their fear of death. But something else changes in them forever. They become incredibly grateful just to be alive. Theology professor Lewis Smedes describes such an event in his book *A Pretty Good Person*. Waking up in a hospital bed after almost dying, he was "seized with a frenzy of gratitude. . . . I blessed the Lord above for the almost unbearable goodness of being alive on this good earth in this good body at this present time."

This prayer by Mary Jean Iron helps me remember not to take small mundane moments for granted:

> Normal day, let me be aware of the treasure you are. Let me learn from you, love you, bless you before you depart. Let me not pass you by in quest of some rare and perfect tomorrow. Let me hold you while I may, for it may not always be so. One day I shall dig my nails into the earth, or bury my face in the pillow, or stretch myself taut, or raise my hands to the sky and want, more than all the world, your return.

What helps are certain attitudes and practices. This list comes from *Attitudes of Gratitude*. These suggestions have deepened the quality of my thankfulness and made expressing gratitude a natural part of my day.

1   Focus on what's right in your life instead of what's wrong.

2   Choose gratefulness "in spite of."

3   Take a moment to say one thing you are thankful for at dinner.

4   Say thank you to others as often as possible.

5   Remember why you love your spouse, kids, and friends.

6   Don't compare your life to others.

7   Give thanks for your body.

8   Practice gratitude daily.

Remember, when it comes to gratitude, as with many other things, it's important to fake it until you make it. I've learned it's precisely when I'm down that I most need to be reminded of anything that's going right.

## Appreciating Age

"Why are we so obsessed with what we lose as we age, and unclear about what we gain?"

—FREDERIC HUDSON

When we talk about gratefulness, what better place to start than by being thankful for our age? Birthdays are good for us; the more we have, the longer we live. Most of us can recite chapter and verse about what's wrong with growing older—sagging skin, less than perfect eyesight, arthritic toes, more pounds, hair growing everywhere except on your head. Or we can be grateful for it all. We've gained in wisdom, understanding, and awareness so much more than we have lost in looks. So like anything else in our lives, we have a choice—to focus on what we've lost or what we've received. One way leads to bitterness, envy, and the perpetual chase for the fountain of youth. The other leads to contentment, satisfaction, and peace of mind.

I was wearing glasses by my third birthday. One of my earliest memories is crawling up in Daddy's lap while he was reading the paper in his red chair and telling him, "Daddy, my eyes twitch." Just in the last few years I've had Lasik surgery three times and cataract surgery. I'm a very visual person and I process almost all information about the world around me through sight. My husband, who has 20/20 vision, asked how come I've never complained about being so dependent on glasses and contacts or all the eye operations. I replied that "the way I see it," the miracle of sight and ophthalmic interventions keep me grateful.

At every moment, you and I have a choice about our reactions. When I find myself bemoaning the ten pounds I've gained, for instance, I immediately stop and send a prayer of thankfulness that I have legs and arms that work. Practicing gratitude allows us to reverse the curse our culture puts on aging. I also remind myself of all the benefits my years have brought me: I'm the person I've always wanted to be. I'd never trade youth for the amazing friends I've cultivated. My family's more together than it's ever been, I'm much easier on myself too. I've become kinder and less critical of myself. I don't sweat the small stuff. I have a deeper connection to God.

For each of us, what we appreciate about aging is different. To get you started thinking about what would go on your list, here are some other thoughts on the benefits of aging:

The Lord blessed the latter end of Job more than the beginning.—*Job 42:12*

The great thing about getting older is that you don't lose all the other ages you've been.—*Madeleine L'Engle*

If we live well, every year we become a year's worth better, smarter, and wiser.—*Molly Ivins*

I used to dread getting older because I thought I would not be able to do all the things I wanted to do, but now that I am older I find that I don't want to do them.—*Nancy Astor*

To be seventy years young is sometimes far more cheerful and hopeful than to be forty years old.
—*Oliver Wendell Holmes Jr.*

Old age is not a disease—it is strength and survivorship, triumph over all kinds of vicissitudes and disappointments, trials and illnesses.—*Maggie Kuhn*

We turn not older with years, but newer every day.
—*Emily Dickinson*

So teach us to number our days, that we may apply our hearts unto wisdom.—*Psalm 90:12*

It is a mistake to regard age as a downhill grade toward dissolution. The reverse is truc. As one grows older, one climbs with surprising strides. —*George Sand*

# Give and You'll Get Back, aka the Boomerang Effect

"It is one of the most beautiful compensations of life that no man can sincerely try to help another without helping himself."

—RALPH WALDO EMERSON

Lillian Carter, mother of President Jimmy Carter, volunteered for the Peace Corps at age sixty-eight and was sent to India for two years. When she returned, Ms. Lillian spent almost two decades lecturing elders not to let age put a limit on their lives. Shortly before her death at age eighty-five she declared, "Sure I'm for helping the elderly. I'm going to be old myself someday."

What Ms. Lillian knew is that helping others can make us feel good about ourselves, keep us fully engaged with another person and feeling needed.

Volunteering increases a person's energy, sense of control over life, and self-esteem. It gives older adults a sense of purpose and meaning that elders who don't reach out to others often lose. A study at Johns Hopkins of older adults volunteering at inner-city schools revealed that while they helped children do better in school, they simultaneously improved their own physical and mental health.

Because being kind and generous also activates the left prefrontal cortex, it has similar positive health effects as optimism and gratitude. For instance, in one large study that tracked twenty-seven hundred people for almost ten years, scientists found that men who did regular volunteer work had death rates two-and-one-half times lower than men who didn't. And in another fascinating study, volunteers who worked directly with those who benefited from their services had a greater immune system boost than the volunteers whose work was restricted to pushing papers at a desk.

The study that is truly amazing, though, when it comes to the physical effects of generosity, is by Harvard researchers showing that giving is such a powerful immune booster that just merely watching someone else in the act of giving works! In this well-known experiment, students looking at a film of Mother Teresa as she tended the sick in Calcutta got a threefold increase in immune function (even those who claimed to dislike Mother Teresa).

I believe strongly that service is the work of the soul. That's why I give my time to antiviolence programs such as the Safe School Summit and the Women's Peace Initiative. If you are angry about drunk drivers you can join me and MADD (Mothers Against Drunk Driving). I also participate in *USA Weekend*'s Make a Difference Day, and when I got fed up with all the trash on TV I became a board member of the Parents Television Council. On the Fourth of July, I return when I can to my hometown of Ashland, Kentucky, for the Judds' Annual Food Drive to help stock the Appalachian Food Pantry.

I'm grateful for my recovery, so one of my biggest volunteer efforts is to help combat hep C. When I was sick, I contacted the American Liver Foundation and was surprised to learn they had only $200,000 in their bank account. I started the Naomi Judd Research and Education Fund with $75,000. Since then I've been able to raise over a million dollars, but we need so much more! The primary goal is to finance research to find a cure for this deadly, mysterious, and highly mutant virus. For example, we awarded one research grant for $100,000 to doctors in Colorado to study pediatric hepatitis C. I can't bear the thought of kids suffering from this condition.

Judd fans and supporters changed my life so drastically for the better. Now I'm very ambitious about giving back. You don't have to have money or even volunteer in a formal way. All you have to do is find ways to GIVE: Generosity In Various Expressions. It can be something as simple as doing five kind things for others a week—bringing soup to a sick friend, helping a grandchild with homework, etc. Scientists have found that these acts really boost your own happiness, especially if you do them all in one day.

So how do you get started? The best way is to think about what you are good at, what talents or skills you have. Are you good at cooking? Perhaps a soup kitchen is right for you. Look also at your interests. What injustice concerns you? What are your unlived dreams? There are plenty of opportunities out there in the world.

If you love travel, consider Friendship Force (www.friendship force.org; 404-522-9490), which is an exchange program in which Americans go to other countries to live with host families and then open their homes to their hosts on a return visit. Love pets? I'll bet my farm the local animal shelter needs you. Believe in peace? Know someone who's experienced domestic violence? There are hundreds of organizations looking for help.

Every Christmas there are local organizations trying to give to needy kids. 'Tis the season for giving. This year, I rode the Santa Train on CSX Railroad through small towns in Appalachia. Santa and I threw out toys and treats from the caboose to hundreds of kids rushing out to the tracks. It made Larry's and my Christmas.

Archbishop Desmond Tutu said, "Do your little bit of good where you are. It is those little bits of good put together that overwhelm the world." Archbishop Tutu, who is battling prostate cancer, not long ago told me that he's enjoying and grateful for every day. Then he grabbed me up to dance in the aisle while Sheryl Crow was performing.

One of the great things about practicing positivism, gratitude, and generosity is that they build on each other. Call it a circle of joy. At Maya Angelou's kitchen table, I asked why she's so outspoken about the importance of generosity. "You shouldn't go through your life with a catcher's mitt on. You'll be happier if you throw something back," she replied.

## Your Turn Now

- Does your attitude need an adjustment? Does looking on the bright side, being grateful and generous, come easily? Or do you feel you need to grow these habits? If you'd like to work on feeling more grateful, commit to the following for three weeks:

    - When things don't go your way, ask yourself, "What could be right about this?"

    - Keep a gratitude journal to write down what you are thankful for each day. Challenge yourself to come up with at least seven things.

- The following affirmation helps me: *What I have, is enough. What I am, is enough. What I do, is enough. What I've achieved, is enough.*

- Find somewhere to give of your time and talents. One resource that can cut down on your legwork to find the right opportunity is www.volunteermatch.org. It is an online matching service where you can type in where you live and what you are interested in doing and they give you a list of organizations that match your request. They have done almost two million referrals so far.

- To donate to the Naomi Judd Research and Education Fund, contact www.liverfoundation.org.

- Join me and millions of other Americans on Make a Difference Day. Make a Difference Day is a celebration of neighbors helping neighbors created by *USA Weekend* magazine. It takes place on the fourth Saturday of every October. It's a fabulous way to do an activity as a family, and if your kids don't appreciate what they have, it could open their eyes. To find out more, go to www.usaweekend.com/diffday.

- Speak positively about yourself and your life: *I'm feeling great! Things are wonderful!* The more positive energy you put out, the more that will come back.

- Do five a day—five kind things, that is. They can include a random act of kindness—feeding someone's parking meter, smiling at strangers, baking cookies for the fire station—or you can be good to the folks nearest and dearest to you: listen without interrupting even if it's hard; pick a bunch of flowers to give to a neighbor. Notice how great you feel and how much better life seems.

- When you talk to yourself, is it in a kind and positive way? Next time you catch yourself being mean or negative to yourself, say something positive out loud: *I'm doing the best I can; I did a great job; I am smart and capable.*

- Look for the hidden blessings in difficult situations. We don't ask for the hardships in our lives, but they always provide opportunities for learning and growth. Hepatitis C helped me rearrange my priorities and simplify my life, and it launched me into a whole new career. When you look at what good came out of a difficulty, you're seeing the divine plan in action and you engage your optimism and hope for facing whatever else may come along.

- What have you gained by aging? What's good about being the age you are? What qualities of heart, mind, and soul have you developed? Make a list of all the good things age has brought you. Then take it out when you're feeling low about that latest wrinkle and read it out loud.

- Dr. Sonja Lyubomirsky of the University of California is a renowned researcher in the field of positive psychology. On my Hallmark show she named eight steps toward a more satisfying life. Some of those steps I've already talked about. Chapter 8 deals with what she's found to be the most important. "Investing time and energy into family and friends. How much money you make, your job title, where you live and even your health don't compare."

"Let your boat be light, packed with only what you need; one or two friends worth the name, someone to love and someone to love you, a cat, a dog . . ."

—JEROME K. JEROME

## 6 | *Stand by Me:* The Importance of Romance, Friendship, and Having Fun

WILL DANCE FOR ROSES. Wy, her husband Roach, Ashley, Larry, and I went to the Indy 500 race to support Ashley's husband Dario as he raced in the largest spectator sport in the world. He took us to the big sponsors' dinner. Lots of money—women were wearing jewels that cost almost as much as a race car. Los Lobos was playing a hip set, but nobody was dancing or really having fun. Wynonna, Ash, and I were swaying together to the rhythm in front of the big shiny empty dance floor. Ashley baited me. "I dare you," she whispered. "What's it worth to you?" I countered. Because she knew I wanted to plant roses across our front fence, she responded, "A hundred dollars' worth of roses."

I agreed just as a middle-aged guy wearing white socks with sandals came over to ask for my autograph. I heard my shy Larry sigh, "Uh-oh, I'm gonna need a drink." I grabbed the fan's arm and pulled him out onto the middle of the dance floor. Elbows began poking sides, pointing and staring. Even Wynonna and Ashley stood there flabbergasted. The willing guy could not have been more of a geek and I was happy to be his geek goddess. I let loose and my new friend, Goober, came up with moves I've never seen a human make, which made it all the more entertaining for everybody. Los Lobos gave us a round of applause. The onlookers soon flooded the floor. (I was just asked to be on ABC's *Dancing with the Stars*. Maybe they saw me dancing?) Ellen DeGeneres says, "There's no one way to dance," and that's kind of my philosophy about everything.

I danced for three reasons. One is that Ashley is the daredevil in our family. She's broken her ankle twice, once horseback riding in our valley and then another time waterskiing in the Outback of Australia. She does her own stunts in movies. For Ashley Judd to taunt me . . . Why, what's a mom to do? I also did it because Wynonna, Ashley, and I can't stand pretentiousness. We often blurt out outrageous things to break the ice and liven things up. Number three: For the Judds, FUN stands for **F**eeling **U**topia **N**ow.

No matter how long you live, life is too short not to enjoy yourself and find as much pleasure as possible in every situation. For most of us, that pleasure is found in love, sex, eating good food, playing sports, friendship, trying new things, and laughing often. Fortunately, these pleasures are good not only for our spirits but our minds and bodies too. Fun has no age limit. My therapist friend Jennie Adams, age seventy-eight, knows more jokes than anyone and gives me really dumb gag gifts that make us both laugh.

# *That Special Someone*

Being in a healthy long-term relationship is definitely one of the biggest delights of getting older. Robert Browning rhapsodized:

> *Grow old along with me!*
> *The best is yet to be,*
> *The last of life, for which the first was made.*

Doesn't it make you ooh and ahh when you see little old couples holding hands? After many years with another person, you don't have to work so hard at your relationship. It's not like the morning after you have sex for the first time, when you're still on trial. You've learned after being through situations together that you can relax. Larry is the best bargain I ever got. To the world you're just one person. But to that one person you are the whole world.

Because Larry and I have been together twenty-six years, we have all kinds of memories that connect us. We're human time machines. We sometimes drive by the little white frame country house where we kissed for the first time in the front yard. We raised Wy and Ashley there under rough conditions and seeing it always brings back bittersweet thoughts. Memories also keep us aware of what's right. It once bugged me the way Larry clanged his spoon against the cereal bowl. When his dad, the Reverend Ralph Strickland, died last year, his family was reminiscing about little things after the funeral. His sister Carole made the noise on her plate and smiled, remembering how their dad always clanged his cereal bowl. Now when Larry clangs, I smile. It's a sweet reminder of a dear man who even performed our marriage ceremony.

The marriage commitment means we continue to grow together. Larry and I have learned to create "sacred space"—a safe atmosphere were we know how to honor, appreciate, and encourage each other. Now intimacy also stands for "into me you see."

A good relationship is like a work of art. And I do mean work! Over the years, we've learned a lot from a relationship therapist. Here are five things that have helped us:

## Keeping Love Alive and the Relationship Working

1    Men and women are wired differently. As John Gray taught, men are from Mars and women from Venus. You must accept the differences rather than being constantly frustrated by them. Understanding the plain facts allows us to give up trying to change them. Information is power and leads to understanding and harmony. I recommend Harville Hendrix's *Getting the Love You Want.* Now if I announce, "Larry, we need to talk," he doesn't automatically want to run into the woods. I'll also ask, "Is this a good time? If not, when?"

2    As Anne Morrow Lindbergh wrote, "The seeds of love must be eternally resown." That means we need to appreciate our partner every day. Don't take him or her for granted. Say "I love you." "Thank you." "Would you please . . . ?" Pay attention when he or she does something well. We need to be the *most* considerate and grateful to the person who is the closest to us.

3  Dr. Phil McGraw himself shared this advice with me. According to him, there's one mistake you can make that's the worst. If you want your relationship to last, don't end an argument by making the other person feel small. If you end a fight with something like "You are so dumb. What was I thinking when I married you?" your relationship is in big trouble. Leave him or her with some semblance of dignity. You don't rupture the possibility for reconnection.

4  Men do want to put their woman up on a pedestal, so keep separate bathrooms if possible, ladies. Just don't be seen grooming. We don't need to be with each other all the time. I've never farted in front of Larry. (I can't say the same for him.)

5  Larry and I have fun together. Sometimes all you can do is laugh—at yourself, your mate, and the places you get stuck. Here are a few chuckles for inspiration:

Errol Flynn died on a seventy-foot boat with a seventeen-year-old girl. Walter has always wanted to go that way, but he's going to settle for a seventeen-footer with a seventy-year-old.
—*Betsy Cronkite, wife of Walter*

When he's late for dinner, I know he's either having an affair or lying dead in the street. I always hope it's the street.
—*Jessica Tandy about her longtime mate, Hume Cronyn*

I told my wife that a husband is like a fine wine; he gets better with age. The next day, she locked me in the cellar.
—*Anonymous*

Tim [Robbins] and I just celebrated seventeen years together, which in Hollywood I think is forty-five. —*Susan Sarandon*

Sexiness wears thin after a while and beauty fades, but to be married to a man who makes you laugh every day, ah . . . now that's a real treat! —*Joanne Woodward*

An archaeologist is the best husband a woman can have; the older she gets, the more interested he is in her.
—*Agatha Christie, whose husband was an archaeologist*

Husbands are like fires. They tend to go out if not taken care of. —*Zsa Zsa Gabor*

The best way to get husbands to do something is to suggest that perhaps they are too old to do it. —*Shirley MacLaine*

If my husband ever leaves me, I'm going with him.
—*Naomi Judd*

Long-term relationships absolutely take work, but they offer such great payoffs when it comes to aging well. Married people live eight years longer on average than those who are single, widowed, or divorced. Part of the reason is that we take better care of ourselves when there is someone around. In studying 27,000 cancer patients, scientists found that single folks died more often because they waited longer to get treated in the first place.

But it's more than that. When they factored in cancer stage and treatment options, married folks *still* did better. Having a partner to talk to, to be supported by, and to care about what happens helps us feel better emotionally. And that translates into positive health benefits by reducing stress hormones and boosting natural killer cells in our immune system. Marriage also decreases depression. Although we sometimes groan, "You're going to drive me crazy," good marriages actually improve mental health. Fortunately, as you will see later in this chapter, single people can reap the same benefits by creating strong friendships and support groups.

## Where to Find Love

If you don't have a special someone right now and want a relationship, don't let age stand in your way. Remember, we're living longer, and people can fall in love at any time in their lives. Lots of people are connecting online. A more old-fashioned way is to get out and do something you love. One of the best places to meet someone who might be right for you is where people come together doing what they love. If you love singing, join a choral group. If it's hiking, join a hiking group. Go by yourself, rather than bringing a friend, so you'll be more likely to strike up a conversation. Consider a special-interest tour or adventure—a yoga week or biking through the Smokies. You can find all kinds of these trips online.

One place many baby boomers are meeting potential mates is at high school or college reunions. They are rekindling old flames with former sweeties who are now divorced or widowed, or connecting to folks they never knew. I've heard of at least a dozen marriages begun at these events.

Besides putting yourself in the right place, you've also got to be in the right frame of mind. Rather than worrying about your bra size or number of wrinkles, focus on the size and condition of your heart. People fall in love with people who are loving. Dr. Judith Orloff, a psychiatrist and practicing intuitive in L.A., explained to me a basic dynamic of energy is that we attract who we are. So the more positive energy we give off, the more we'll draw to ourselves. In her book *Positive Energy*, Judith writes that "this human form of ours is a subtle energy transmitter. We're constantly sending out signals which others on similar frequencies pick up on and gravitate towards." A sex addict can walk into a bar and quickly spot a fellow sexaholic. Our relationship with ourselves is reflected in the relationships we have with others.

Love yourself first. Then come from love, not fear. Rather than worrying, "Does he like me? Am I going to be rejected again?" think, "I need to understand I'm worthy and unique." Then, "How can I be caring to this person? What can I give?" Rather than waiting to be invited, invite someone to do something. Here's how Susan Jeffers puts it in her book *Dare to Connect*: "Don't warm yourself by the fire; be the one to light it!" But then above all, don't measure your worthiness by whether someone is interested in you or not.

If you're coming from a sense of desperation or suffer from low self-esteem, your first action should be the favor of some self-healing. Others will treat you the way you've trained them to treat you. Jeffers's book is good. So is Sue Patton Thoele's *The Courage to Be Yourself.* Or try therapy or a support group. We attract what we feel worthy of.

## Come On, Grandpa, Light My Fire

"When it comes to sex, the most important six inches are the ones between the ears."

—DR. RUTH WESTHEIMER

Ever notice the number of jokes that make fun of old folks' sexual drive or ability? Here are some funny definitions:

**Old is when . . .**

"getting a little action" means you don't need to take fiber today.

"getting lucky" means finding your car in the parking lot.

"an all-nighter" means not having to get up to pee in the night.

As those jokes reveal, people assume the sex drive dwindles away after we pass the age for procreation. That just ain't so. Research shows that 50 percent of people in their fifties have sex at least once a week and 30 percent in their seventies do—and most folks in their fifties, sixties, and seventies report wanting it more frequently. Sex as we age is different, that's all, just like everything else. Do you think the way you did at twenty? I hope not! Ditto for having sex. The intensity can still be there. The frequency may or may not be. In other words, it's not about quantity, it's about quality.

Sex is a very important part of an intimate relationship. It's an exchange of energy that makes us feel good emotionally as well as physically. It creates stronger connections between a couple. We have 5 million touch receptors in our skin, 3,000 per fingertip. Our bodies are meant to touch and be touched. (Older folks are often starved for touch. That's why every time I visit a nursing home, I offer hugs.) As we age, sex may require more communication and humor, both of which can actually bring us closer together.

It's also good for our bodies. During sex, the body produces 200 percent more endorphins than average. Sex reduces mild depression, eliminates headaches—there goes that old excuse—and is ten times more effective than Valium in producing a calm, relaxed state.

A Scottish study even found that sex makes you look younger— those having sex four to five times a week look more than ten years younger than those doing it twice a week. They're not sure why but think that the testosterone released during orgasm helps keep men's muscle mass and the surge of estrogen that women have during sex may help skin stay youthful and hair shiny. *All My Children* soap star Ruth Warrick, who worked until her death at eighty-eight, credited her youthful vigor to an active sex life, including numerous relationships after the age of sixty-five. How's that for inspiration?

You've probably seen my friend Dr. Mehmet Oz on *Oprah*. He claims that "the average woman thinks about sex every two to three days, while the average man thinks about sex at least once a day." If you aren't feeling the urge at all or aren't having sex as often as you want to, the problem is most likely physical.

One thing to consider is how fit you are. People who work out regularly have more and better sex. Getting the blood flowing benefits all our body parts. So does eating right, limiting alcohol, and quitting smoking (see Chapter 8). Talk to your doctor about the kinds of medications you're taking. Lots of prescription drugs can interfere with sexual health.

You might have your testosterone level checked by blood specimen since it is a sex hormone in both men and women. Low levels can result in lack of sexual desire, lack of strong orgasms, and impaired potency. Both men and women have biological clocks that lower hormone levels as time passes. In women, these changes ultimately result in menopause. But it happens in men too; it's just less obvious. A man's testosterone level drops about 1 percent a year starting at thirty. That means by age seventy-four, it's dropped 44 percent. When men have low testosterone, they're not only going to have a low sex drive, but they're not going to have to shave as often. They may feel listless or depressed, have trouble sleeping, or experience muscle weakness.

Dry Vagina Monologues? There are over-the-counter lubricants. Women can also be prescribed a topical testosterone ointment that you apply on your skin a couple of times a week to stimulate libido. Warning: Using too much can cause temporary hair loss. Men who need a testosterone boost may also be prescribed shots, pills, topical gels, or patches.

Of course, for men there is also the Viagra solution. If you are thinking of that route, don't just order it online. See a qualified physician who can test you for heart problems, diabetes, and low testosterone. Male health specialists claim that Viagra is being overprescribed and is masking other problems that should be addressed. (P.S. Are you as angry as I am that Viagra is covered by insurance and birth control pills aren't?)

No matter your age or relationship status, you are a sexual being. Remember what the famous sexologist Alex Comfort said: Having sex is like riding a bike. It takes a bit of work and balance, is good for your health, and a hell of a lot of fun. My pal Dr. Andrew Weil has a fabulous book, *Healthy Aging*. He addresses how important touch is throughout life. Dr. Weil says that if you are alone, self-stimulation is always an option. (Isn't that what's meant by "Sisters Are Doing It for Themselves"?) Dr. Weil considers it a healthy practice throughout life. He also acknowledges that for some people, diminishing interest in sex can be liberating and a welcome change.

# Together, We're Happier and Healthier

"A faithful friend is the medicine of life and immortality."
—ECCLESIASTES 6:16

Are you aware of the Power of We? No matter our age, we all need a variety of friends—old friends who've known us forever, who bore witness at our dad's memorial service or watched us struggle through divorces; friends who are wise and can offer us advice when we're stuck; friends who are great at boosting us up when we're down; friends who know how to listen when we need to rant, can find us a specialist, help us move, or get a date for a social event; friends we can introduce our mate to knowing they won't try to steal him. If you're in a couple, you also need couple friends—people to have fun with along with your spouse. And we need friends of all ages so that we don't get too cut off from other generations. I absolutely love hanging with my daughters and their coterie of "hens."

Nothing can take the place of a pal who's been around through all our stuff. Someone who knew our parents and siblings and "gets" us. I'm fortunate that even though I don't live in my hometown, I travel a lot, so I get to check in with childhood pals. Growing up in Ashland, Kentucky, Pat Bailey Fornash and I were in each other's homes and walked to school together. Now she's a teacher for the magnet school in Lexington. Recently, after a speaking gig in Lexington, I spent the day with Pat catching up. Our common bond of beliefs and values from being raised the same way allows us to still be compatible as adults fifty years later. We both cried when it came time for me to climb on my bus and leave. George Herbert was right: "The best mirror is an old friend."

Old friends are our link to the past. Unlike new friends, we've borne witness to each other's origins and already been through a lot together. I went to my fortieth high school reunion with my first boyfriend, Randy Memmer, and his wife, Kay. In the third grade, Randy and I used to scale the fence at the National Guard Armory and play army in the tanks. He gave me his father's dog tags (of course, my mother made me give them back). Driving to the reunion, I nervously confided to Randy I was going to be crushed if any of our classmates called me Naomi. They all knew me as Diana. Not one did. No one asked for my autograph either, not even for their kid's piano teacher. It was such a relief they weren't starstruck. Whew! The older we get, the more we each long to feel truly known.

Reunions are an interesting barometer of how well others your chronological age are handling aging. My buddies Pam Dixon and Jennifer Day, like Pat, never have had plastic surgery and look much like they did in high school. Their exuberant personalities still make them immensely likable. As Proverbs 27:19 states: "A mirror reflects a man's face, but what he really is like is shown by the kind of friends he chooses."

Larry and I gathered a group of five couples our age dubbed "The World According to Us." We have a lot in common. At our holiday dinner party, I purposefully separated husbands and wives. I seated half our guests at the dining room table and half at the kitchen table. In the dining room, I posed serious questions like: "You're head of immigration. Which would you allow into the country—people who were desperate for refuge or people who'd won a Nobel Prize and could greatly increase the quality of life here?" You find out a lot about character real fast and stimulate lively debate. When you consider others' opinions, you expand your own thinking. Meanwhile, Larry was in charge of the kitchen crowd. They were howling with laughter, telling jokes and wild stories. What a contrast!

Like love relationships, friendships are essential to happy, healthy aging. I'll cite a couple of studies to help get you off the couch and out meeting new people or reconnecting with the friends you already have. Seventeen thousand people in Sweden between twenty-nine and seventy-four were studied for six years. Those with the fewest social ties were almost four times as likely to die, despite age or physical health. Three thousand people in the United States were studied for nine to twelve years. Men with fewer connections to others had two to three times the disease rates of cancer, heart disease, and stroke as men with strong friendships. If you look only at cardiovascular disease, the risks from lack of friends are as strong as smoking, obesity, high cholesterol, lack of exercise, or drinking too much alcohol.

The Nurses' Health Study shows the same thing—having close friends and/or relatives results in greater health and happiness in the women studied. You even have fewer colds with more friends. Another study showed that you only need four real friends to reap the longevity effects of social ties. You need a minimum of seven social contacts per week to keep mental health.

The image of Aunt Bee and Clara languidly gossiping at the kitchen table in Mayberry isn't likely today. My close friend Dorthey lives down the road in a double-wide trailer and we've seen each other several times a week for the past sixteen years. We know everything about each other. And I do mean everything, because we see each other so often.

If there's a bond you've let lapse, you can pick up whenever and wherever you left off. For instance, Tina Nova, PhD, lives and works in biotechnology in Southern California. We met years ago when she devised the PSA test for men's prostrate cancer detection. She's currently going through a divorce, and today I received a three-page letter describing the autopsy on the death of her marriage. As an intellectual, Tina processes thoughts and feelings in a unique manner. Writing down her emotions helps her untangle them. Tina's been reading *Naomi's Breakthrough Guide.* She wrote that it's like I'm sitting right there with her at her kitchen table as she reads my writing. I'm no intellectual, but I'm grateful for the many different ways friendships help us feel we're not alone and that someone really cares how we're doing.

Psychologists who study resilience are interested in some people's ability to thrive even in very difficult circumstances. As we've seen, resilience has partly to do with having an optimistic outlook and the habit of practicing gratitude. What scientists have also found is that it's about the ability to look for the most health-giving people anywhere and connect to them. Resilient souls find friends who are good for them no matter what is going on in their lives. New towns, job challenges, a serious illness—resilient people find others to connect to and help them.

Researchers also say that women tend to live longer than men partly because they are more social. Men tend to find themselves lost when their wives die because they've put all their eggs in one basket and made all of their social connections to one person.

Part of why it's easier for women is biological. Researchers at UCLA found that the stress response in women is different from that in men. It used to be believed that when people experience stress, they trigger hormones that alert the body to fight, freeze, or run like hell. What these scientists discovered is that women have another response—tending and befriending. Under stress, our bodies also produce oxytocin, a hormone that encourages us to tend to children and gather with other women. Guess that explains why we even go to the powder room together!

Are you resilient? Do you reach out to others when times are tough? Man or woman, if this is not your tendency, for the sake of your well-being as you get older, you need to learn how to create and maintain friendships. Here's a tip from Dale Carnegie: "You can make more friends in two months by becoming interested in other people than you can in two years by trying to get other people interested in you." Reach out and touch someone—the life you keep may be your own.

## Furry Friends

"It's funny how dogs and cats know the inside of folks better than other folks do, isn't it?"
—ELEANOR H. PORTER

I have animal attraction—I *love* my pets. I didn't completely grasp the power of pets until I started touring on the bus with Banjo, my dog. It gets lonely on the road, and he gave me a sense of home. Banjo was somebody to come back to while Larry stayed on the farm. Pets are stress busters too. They can help you press the "paws" button. Banjo was also an icebreaker. Dressed down, I would walk him in the afternoons when we were performing. People didn't recognize me and would come up and chat because of Banjo.

When I was bedridden with hepatitis C and emotionally bereft, the constancy and cuddly furry warm body of my little creature offered such "creature" comfort. Dogs smile with their tails. For them, life is a ball.

Pets like Banjo become family members. Psychologists have known for a long time that pets can make us feel better about being alive by reducing depression and easing loneliness. But pets not only lift our spirits but help us heal faster from surgery, control diabetes, lower blood pressure, and recover faster from heart attacks. Now they're not only man's best friend, but healers too.

*Any* furry pet will do. That's why many nursing homes invite pet visitors—dogs, cats—to brighten residents' moods and bolster immune systems.

What about you? Do you enjoy the companionship a pet can provide?

# Pardon Me, But Is Your Rut Showing?

"The aging process has you firmly in its grasp if you never get the urge to throw a snowball."

—DOUG LARSON

Experts who study centenarians have another message for you—make sure you continue to be curious and try new things. It used to be that aging was thought of as a process of steadily disengaging—you did less, saw fewer and fewer people, took fewer risks, and cared less about virtually everything except your bowel movements. Now they believe that many of the symptoms we associated with aging—declining mental and physical abilities—are *caused* by disengaging, not the other way around. The more we push our own self-imposed limits of what we think we're capable of doing, the longer, healthier, and happier we'll get to stick around. It will even help us lose weight, according to one study. Researchers who asked folks to do something different every day—listen to a new radio station, for instance—found that they lost and kept off weight. No one is sure why, but scientists speculate that getting out of routines makes us more aware in general.

But it takes action to break out of ruts. Scientists tell us that 99 percent of our daily lives are lived in habit—what we eat, do, see, and say from the time we wake up to the moment our head hits the pillow again. Routines are easy and comfortable, but they also deaden us. When we break out of our ruts and take a risk, we feel more alive, more mentally awake, and more aware of our environment. I go to bookstores frequently and will purchase magazines that are outside my politics or interests just to challenge my beliefs and keep my mind fresh.

I know a woman in her eighties who has been practicing risk taking for the past ten years. "I make sure to do at least one daring thing for my birthday," she explained. "One year a young friend took me on a motorcycle ride. The next year he took me to a Rolling Stones concert. I've also climbed mountains, been snorkeling at night, gone skinny-dipping. I do have to keep my adventures from my kids and grandkids. They wouldn't think these adventures are 'appropriate.' But I know that if I don't keep expanding and stretching, my life will just get smaller and shrink. I've seen it happen to too many friends."

What risk are you willing to take right now? To inspire you, consider Jeanne Calment, the oldest person in the world who died in 1997 at 122. She took up fencing at eighty-four. Fencing! Other rut breakers, as reported by gerontologist Walter M. Bortz II: the man who bungee-jumped 210 feet for his hundredth birthday, the one-hundred-year-old woman who took up dance classes, the 103-year-old guy who started playing golf at ninety-two and recently shot a ninety-eight.

I stay open to new experiences (besides sweeping strangers onto dance floors) by attending conferences on topics of personal interest like integrative medicine, public speaking, art, and social issues. (To find them, check out your newspaper and magazine ads.) I take in new ideas and make diverse connections. When I'm there, I feel like Elijah and

Grace at an amusement park: What ride are we gonna try next? I get such a rush of feel-good hormones that I feel high.

You don't have to bungee-jump or speak in front of a thousand people. Pick something new that's appealing, like singing (one of my favorites, as you might imagine). Seniors who sing visit the doctor less often and have less depression, less need for medicine, and fewer falls and other injuries. Or take up canasta—group games have been found to be a great exercise for stress reduction. It really doesn't matter what the activity is as long as you enjoy it. As poet Phyllis McGinley said, "A hobby a day keeps the doldrums away."

## What's So Funny?

"He who laughs, lasts!"
—MARY PETTIBONE POOLE

If laughter can be considered internal jogging, I am a laughaholic 'cause I want to stay in shape. As a hillbilly from Kentucky, I offer the following for your internal workout:

### Hillbilly Medical Terms

- Morbid: a higher offer
- Impotent: distinguished or well-known
- GI series: soldier ball games
- Barium: what doctors do when patients die
- Outpatient: the patient fainted
- Terminal illness: getting sick at the airport

- Tumor: more than one
- Organic: a church musician

The average adult laughs just fifteen times a day. No one's put a number on how often children laugh, but anyone who's been around kids knows that it's a lot more than *fifteen* times! Somehow, growing up creates hardening of the funny bone in some old geezers.

Laughter is to our soul as soap is to our bodies. It cleanses us. It's also like an instant vacation, as Milton Berle said. Studies prove that folks who appreciate humor are less stressed. That's because humor helps us dodge life's arrows and keeps us from taking ourselves or our circumstances too seriously. It also can help solve problems by encouraging us to think of our situation in a different way. If you're a joker, say scientists, you are more likely to be more confident, have more friends, and feel less stress than more serious types. Every time we see each other, singer Vince Gill and I have a "joke-off." As of now, Vince knows more jokes than anyone.

Laughter is good medicine. It raises blood pressure just slightly and increases the quantity of oxygen we take in and carbon dioxide we breathe out. When we laugh, various muscles throughout our bodies tense and then relax the same way as when you do yoga. This helps us stay limber physically as well as emotionally. Laughing for ten minutes is as strenuous as rowing a hundred strokes! And guess what—laughing decreases stress hormones in your bloodstream and releases the specific feel-good hormones that increase mental alertness. It also strengthens your immune system by increasing the number of natural killer cells. The health effects are so positive that in India, there are even laughing clubs where people get together to laugh on purpose.

A sense of humor eased my grim struggle with hepatitis C, as well as the other challenges in my life. I'd shock people by requesting liver and onions for dinner or by asking for Carter's Little Liver Pills. I paid attention when Norman Cousins reported that he healed his crippling arthritis not only with traditional medicine, but by watching the Marx Brothers and the Three Stooges as well. Here's how Dr. Clifford Kuhn of the University of Louisville School of Medicine put it: "If medicine could harness the proven health benefits of laughter, drug companies would be knocking themselves out to get the patent."

Take the words of comedian Michael Pritchard to heart: *"You don't stop laughing because you grow old. You grow old because you stop laughing."*

## Your Turn Now

- If you are in a relationship, what can you do to add a bit of romance? A candlelit dinner? Dress up and go out like when you were dating? A chick flick? (Studies have shown that such movies increases a man's sexy feelings more than an action movie, even if he complains about watching it.)

- Go see Rob Becker's *Defending the Caveman,* a hysterical one-man act about why hairy-legged men are the way they are. It will not only give you a laugh, but also some perspective on the differences between men and women.

- If you don't have a sweetie pie, try reading *How Not to Stay Single After 40* by Nita Tucker. It's a very positive book with lots of great suggestions. If you choose to enter the world of online dating, realize that the big ones—match.com, eharmony, Yahoo! Personals, and American Singles—offer the most candidates, but

you have to go through a lot of frogs to find your prince.
Try narrowing your search through a niche site, like
www.bigchurch.com for Christians or www.mycountry
match.com for country music lovers. Go to Google and put in
your interest group followed by the words "online dating." Like
"pet lovers online dating." Chances are there's something. (Yes,
datemypet.com.)

- Do you have a strong social network? Do you have a friend you
  can call for advice? If you were sick, would there be someone
  you could call for help? How about to enjoy a movie with? If
  not, how can you create more social support—join a club or a
  church, start an activity in your community? One woman who
  moved to a new town to be closer to her daughter bemoaned the
  lack of a current events class. So she started one—and made
  several new friends in the process.

- Start an Aging Gratefully group in your town. Go to lunch
  once a week or more. Find some folks who want to support
  one another in thinking positively, living on purpose, getting
  out of ruts, and staying fit mentally and physically. And laughing a lot.

- Do you need an animal in your life? An adoption from a local
  animal shelter is a great way to go. If you don't have the space for
  a dog or cat, consider a bird or a fish. I enjoy my goldfish so
  much that I wrote a children's book, *Gertie the Goldfish and the
  Christmas Surprise.* One grandma I know had breakfast each
  morning with her canaries eating off her plate and actually got
  them to lay eggs.

- List twenty-five things you've always had a hankering to do. Pick one and create a plan to make it happen in the next three months. Break the plan into smaller chunks if need be. (Before you decide to climb Mount Everest, for instance, pick a hill in your hometown.) When you've done one, choose another item. Use your birthday to add to or revise your list. It's okay to change your mind. If you're no longer interested in hang gliding, cross it off.

- Consider a cruise, or attend a class or seminar on a subject of interest.

- One way around the limits we set for ourselves is to imagine you will live until at least ninety. If you're fifty and take up the guitar today, at ninety you will have been playing forty years!

- Need a good laugh? Rent a funny video or go to www.get amused.com, the largest joke bank online. Or start an email joke exchange with friends who are far away. Get Gary Larsen's or Jeff Foxworthy's cartoon books—my personal favorites.

"If you ever start feeling like you have the goofiest, craziest, most dysfunctional family in the world, all you have to do is go to a state fair. Because after five minutes at the fair, you'll be going, 'You know, we're all right. We are dang near royalty.' "
—JEFF FOXWORTHY

## 7 | *Terms of Endearment:* Getting Along with Children, Grandchildren, and Parents

(aka *Rosemary's Baby, Alien, War and Peace, Psycho, Meet the Parents, Trading Places, A Time to Kill, The Bad Seed, The Usual Suspects*)

I WAS LOUNGING in a comfy chair on Ashley's veranda watching Wy and her husband Roach play Elijah and Grace at badminton. As the sun was setting, fireflies began to twinkle. Ashley's roses were in full bloom and lusciously fragrant. We'd just had supper and were feeling full and content. It was an exquisitely ordinary family event—three generations enjoying a summer's eve and one another. Larry and I looked at each other silently wishing, Could we just freeze-frame this moment? Would it tear a hole in the universe?

Of course in our family, like yours, it's not all lemonade and enchanting evenings. We hold fast to these peaceful scenes to remind us of what it should be like next time there's a spat. In reality, the only difference between our family and yours is that, unfortunately, everything that goes on between us is broadcast around the world in salaciously exaggerated form. For instance, the last time all three of us were on *Oprah*, Wy named a few ways they felt I'd failed as a mom. Although my book *Naomi's Breakthrough Guide* had been out for six months, Ashley had never even mentioned it to me. Until, that is, that moment on national TV. Suddenly she was telling Oprah about how good she thought the book was, as if I wasn't sitting there next to them. She couldn't acknowledge it while we were taking a walk to the lake the week before? Nope. Spit it out on *Oprah*. If you happened to have seen that show, you now know why I started to cry. I also have learned that I, in various ways over the years, have unintentionally contributed to her not being able to tell me in another way and time, and have been working very hard on changing that.

No one pushes our buttons more than family. Heck, they installed them! That's because with closeness comes conflict. (If I say something in the woods and Wy and Ashley aren't there to hear me, am I still wrong?) As our children become adults, we need to find new ways of relating to them. Then, when they become parents, we have to figure out how to establish connections to our precious grandchildren. A lot of us baby boomers have the added task of dealing with our own elderly parents while simultaneously trying to maintain this communication and connection to the two younger generations. Aging parents can require a great deal of our time. In the meantime, throw in the complex trick of how to maintain our marriage and personal life.

I believe strongly that one of the keys to aging gratefully is learning how to stay close to our loved ones. They are an intense microcosm of the rest of the world around us. My own family is my greatest source of joy as well as frustration. They are the folks who know me best, love me best, and are there for me no matter what. We make each other laugh the hardest, scream the loudest, and cry the deepest. Agony and ecstasy. It's what keeps therapists in business.

Living in a vacuum sucks (pun intended). Researchers have discovered that close family connections help us stay healthy in mind and body as we grow older. The long-lived Okinawans have the saying, "One cannot live in this world without the support of others," and they rely very much on close family members as part of what they call their "connecting circle." While I sometimes moan, "You'll be the death of me," a Harvard study discovered that close family relationships, along with marriage and friends, helped people live two to three times longer over a nine-year period than those without, regardless of physical health, age, gender, or lifestyle choices.

There are new proven therapeutic negotiations that can teach you how to have healthy relationships so that you'll have your family's love and care to rely on your whole life. You may be the parent, but at some point you will have to look at your children as your equal in order to understand them. And if we open our hearts and minds, we'll have a readymade place to offer all of our own love and wisdom to. George Vaillant, the lead researcher of the Harvard Study of Adult Development, summed it up after studying hundreds of individuals over fifty years: "It is poverty in love, not poverty in dollars, that makes all the difference in old age."

That's why I keep hanging in there with my family, trying to stay current by learning all I can from our family therapist. Are you like me— the best of intentions, heart full of pure love? Oh, but that's not enough. I also need good communication techniques.

## Ties That Bind

"The family is the country of the heart."
—GIUSEPPE MAZZINI

One of the greatest challenges of many families is that we're often geographically dispersed. Because Wy, Ashley, and I travel so much for work, we've deliberately chosen to live down the road from one another. When we are at home, we're close by. I can literally feel when they're there. It gives me great comfort. Plus I can see the grandkids. The kids know where the key to my door is hidden and have clothes, toys, books, etc., at my house.

Wy and Ashley are often not home, so it helps me to be able to visualize where they are. Having been to the places Wynonna plays, I can easily follow her in my mind: I know that arena and I know the hotel. I know she's going to go on stage at eight and I even know some of the fans who are probably out by the bus. That's why I try to visit Ashley on her movie sets—so I can see her in her world.

Do you know how your kids and grandkids spend their time? Unless you make an effort to see your family on a regular basis, particularly if you have married children you must share with the in-laws, years can go by between events such as weddings, funerals, and graduations. Staying connected takes work. So you need to be responsible for creating opportunities.

Some families try staying plugged in by taking annual vacations together—parents, children, and grandchildren. If you can't physically be together, there are plenty of creative ways to love across distance. You can exchange books, DVDs, and music with kids or grandkids. Record yourself reading an age-appropriate book and send it to your grandchild. Send a phone card that they can use to call you. Share their interests—if it's rafting they love, consider inviting them on a rafting trip. Teach them something you know—one grandma started knitting a poncho and then sent it to her eight-year-old granddaughter to continue. When the young one got stuck, she sent it back to Grandma to finish. Now the granddaughter's wearing what they created together.

Because we're often in different time zones, I have a mom line—a phone that's for Wy and Ashley only, to call me any time, twenty-four hours a day. If it rings, I answer. Besides the phone to stay connected (I don't do email), I get duplicate prints made of photos and cut out pictures of family members' heads. I select a magazine with lots of pictures of people in funny situations like someone getting knighted. Then I paste the little head on it and send it to them. For instance, I found a picture of Sean Connery dressed in a kilt, and since Dario is Scottish as well, I put his head on it. I placed it in a care package to Ashley and she got a big kick out of it, passing it around to everybody on the movie set.

Wy called me from backstage at the Apollo in New York where she was performing. Grace had just had a swimming accident, and since I live so close by, I was able to rush over and ride in the ambulance with her. A few weeks later, Larry and I took her and Elijah to a pottery place in Franklin, where they decorated and signed a large platter in appreciation to the guys in the rescue squad. Not being around our grandkids would be like reading a book with some important chapters missing.

Ever notice the word *kindred?* Do you suppose it means "dread of kin who overstay their welcome"? When you have adult children, sometimes it's your responsibility, if you are able, to go where they are. But come often and leave soon. Try to remember they're in the midst of their lives like you were when you were their age. Larry reminds me of that all the time, which helps me not take it personally when I don't see my girls as often as I might want. I have to tell myself they're not mad and it's not that they don't love me. It's just that they're pretty consumed with their own lives.

It also helps if you remember what your mind-set was when you were their age, but then try to resist making the comparison ("Well, when I was your age . . ."). That reminds me of the joke where the guy says, "Well, when I was your age, son, I was walking to school uphill both ways in the snow barefoot," and the kid says, "Well, when Abraham Lincoln was your age, he was president." It's all relative.

Some family members will also create unnecessary emotional distance by making assumptions about family members based on the past—oh, she's always been controlling, he's irresponsible and self-centered, she's the ambitious one. She's too introverted to come to a family holiday. He's a workaholic and always too busy. Outmoded beliefs create walls. People do change and assumptions stand in the way of being current with one another. There's a very simple solution to this tendency—ask. Would you like to come to the picnic? How are you feeling about your job? What can I do to help? Asking a question with genuine curiosity not only brings us up to date but also strengthens the connection between us. (While you're at it, don't forget the power of a sincere compliment!) Parents are notorious for causing adult siblings to relapse into childhood patterns.

One of the hardest but most effective things I've learned being a mother and grandmother is when to keep my mouth shut. A closed mouth gathers no foot. That's particularly tricky in our circumstances. As celebrities, my girls and I don't have a lot of people around us who will call us on our stuff or confront us in any way about anything negative. This is pretty much true for all celebrities. It comes with the territory. So sometimes Larry and I feel like we're the only ones who can tell our girls something straight up, and we've asked them to do the same for us. It's all about timing, though. Knowing when to speak and when to bite my tongue is one of my greatest challenges. I've got the bite marks to prove it! (What's the difference between a smart parent and a wise one? The smart one knows what to say, the wise one knows whether or not to say it.) A good rule of thumb: Talk less, hug more.

## Strong Boundaries and Low Expectations

"No matter how old a mother is, she watches her middle-aged children for signs of improvement."

—FLORIDA SCOTT-MAXWELL

Author Victoria Secunda explains the mother-daughter relationship this way: "A daughter is a mother's gender partner, her closest ally in the family confederacy, an extension of herself. And mothers are their daughters' role model, their biological and emotional road map, the arbiter of all their relationships." As a consequence, things can get messy as mothers and daughters try to find new footing as adults.

If the mother-daughter relationship isn't already hard enough, the fact that I raised Wy and Ashley as a single parent and we're all three now in the public eye makes our relationship ridiculously intense. That's why we like to take advantage of a very wise counselor.

However well intentioned, even a sincere desire to tell my offspring (or sprung-offs, as I like to call them) something I believe will help them can still be perceived as a form of manipulation. Our counselor likened it to me telling them something affirming and loving while they're wearing headphones. They don't hear what I'm saying, because they're listening to a negative tape from the past. I now try to honor their adulthood and their right to their own timeline and path.

Before you can be real with others or be your higher self, you must first heal the wounds of your own past. It's critical for you to be aware of how your unconscious acting out of past roles is affecting you today. People who hurt hurt other people. Being stuck in old behavior and thought patterns decreases your ability to see the present clearly. Is your own past still so alive it's draining your efforts to be fully in the now? Use your memories instead of letting them continue to use you.

If you're willing to take time to look at your past with your kids in a forward-thinking way using solution-oriented techniques with a therapist, amazing progress can be made. Just keep showing up with an open mind.

Here are a couple of ideas that can help parents and their adult children open up to seeing each other in a much better light: (1) Be willing to acknowledge that the contributions each one makes to the relationship are valid. Know that relationships are a fifty-fifty process and each person must be responsible for his or her own 50 percent. (2) Use reflective listening. This is where the other person makes a statement to you and you repeat it back exactly. You don't interpret or respond. You allow the other to truly feel heard. When we are listened to, that honest attention is a magnet. It draws us closer. We don't feel judged or censored and we begin to feel safe. Reflective listening, the practice of repeating the other person, teaches us how to be better listeners. Your child will be more willing to talk with you because she will feel safe. In return you both will communicate better because you will feel heard.

When there's a disagreement, can you get out of your rational mind and let go of what you think happened or what you think is right or wrong? You need to start with a beginner's mind. Remember, the old ways of thinking and acting aren't working, so be willing at least to act as if you know nothing.

Being completely open-minded will shock people. They will be totally thrown off. You're no longer acting like the person they're convinced you are. It will rock their world. Shift happens! Once after a therapy session, the girls looked at me, puzzled, and asked, "Who are you and what have you done with our mom?"

Come up with code words to immediately identify old triggers for past conflicts. If I start to talk too much about my TV show, the girls will say a secret phrase to stop me.

Develop the habit of saying therapeutic phrases like:

- Is this a good time to talk about this?

- Would you like to know what I think about that?

- Are you open to a suggestion?

- That's not my reality, but tell me why you feel that way.

- What is it that you want from me right now?

Over the years, we've developed among us a number of unspoken rules to encourage that separateness. They might just have a ring of familiarity to you too. One is that you're not allowed to ask why your daughter makes the choices she does. Or what she's doing when. Wy and Ashley want me to be Mom and not have to share me with the public. They can come to my house and go through everything because they feel it's still their home. But I can't even look through a stack of books on a coffee table in their homes without raising suspicions that I'm snooping. Some things will never change no matter how much therapy you go through. And of course it is never good to make comments on a daughter's clothing, weight, makeup, friends, parenting, or grooming.

One of the great things about aging is the wisdom we've gained through experience. I now know, for example, that any time the three of us Judds get together, there's potential for conflict. We're a mob of emotions. So when I find myself worrying in advance about a get-together, I remember that I cannot control anything about another human being, including my two girls. In fact, there is only one thing I can control—myself. I can only change myself. I can hope that others change, I can encourage, I can support, but I will never change or control them.

I used that wisdom recently when reuniting the family after Ashley had been away for months on a movie set. I so wanted Ashley to have a lovely evening. Being vigilant about what I can and can't control, I reminded myself I couldn't be responsible for Ashley's expectations or her feelings. But I could get in touch with my own expectations and fears.

Once I identified those, I thought to myself, "Okay, what would I do if . . . ?" I played out every contingency and decided in advance how I would respond. I figured out my boundaries. Then I felt better. I showed up relaxed and in the mood to enjoy myself.

Boundaries exist to protect us from taking abuse. They tell others their actions are violating the integrity of our personal truth. Good boundaries make close families. We need to make clear to our relatives how we want to be treated. Just because we are swimming in the same gene pool doesn't mean I can assume anything. And we need to decide in advance what we're going to do if we're being mistreated. When you figure it out beforehand—I'm leaving if they start making fun of me—you're more likely to do it calmly and therefore cause less harm. You don't have to cause a ruckus, or blame or shame anyone. You just get out of harm's way. Move before it hits the fan and you don't get any on you.

I value taking responsibility for the past. I've been honest with my daughters about the mistakes I made raising them and about things I wish I had done differently. But after I owned up to my mistakes, that's it. The two of them are grown women now and the statute of limitations on blame is over. I firmly believe in the old saying that after thirty you can't blame your parents anymore. That was then. This is now. And you have the advantage of being able to expose yourself to psychological truths and therapies. You must take responsibility for your tomorrow. That goes for me—and for them.

Another crucial key in getting along with adult children is being able to let go of your own expectations. Conflict arises when the other person doesn't meet your expectations. I'm an idealist. I'm so Donna Reed. I just want everybody to have a lovely meal. I want the weather to be good so we can be out on the screened-in porch. I want, I want, I want. The more I let go of wanting and accept the reality of what's actually happening, the happier I am.

When you let go of expectations, you make room for whatever happens. As adults, we need to relinquish our fantasy of our parents. My mother was never one to give compliments, and I always wanted them from her. I've had to learn to give up my "fantasy mom." Recently she called and left a message. She announced, "I watched you do your speaking engagement tonight and I felt very proud of you." Then she chuckled and added, "P.S. I know this has been a long time coming. Now there you have it. Love, your mom." Better late than never.

# My Full Truth Is Still Only Half the Whole Story

"Honor God by accepting each other, as Christ has accepted you."
—ROMANS 15:7

One of the smartest things we can do with every family member is to really see him or her as a unique individual. That's huge. One of the big mistakes we make is assuming that because they are related to us, they are just like us. Nope.

I realized that recently when I was visiting Ashley at her home after not seeing her for months. Her hair and wardrobe people were there working on her because she had a very important photo shoot to do the next day. We had supper together and the entourage moved into her bathroom. Samantha was showing her dozens of outfits, Theresa was doing her hair while Ashley was reading her script, and I was sitting on the floor watching. After about an hour and a half, Ashley whispered to me, "I really need my space, Mom," which was my cue to leave. Ashley knows her boundaries. She was frustrated at having arrived home only to be surrounded by people. If I had said that to my mother at any age, I would have gotten a jar of pickles poured over my head (which she actually did one time—a whole jar of sticky syrupy sweet pickles).

I didn't get upset at being asked to leave because I've come to realize that Ashley and I are very different. Our upbringing couldn't be more different. If I were in a situation where I thought my mom was the extra person in the room when I was feeling claustrophobic, I would tolerate it by going within, centering myself, and breathing deeply. On the other hand, I raised Ashley to speak up for herself and express her needs. We've worked hard to learn to speak our truth to one another.

Maybe someday I can have this kind of relationship with my mom. Or maybe I should just relinquish my "fantasy mom." Gotcha!

It's crucial to understand that we each have our own reality. Our truth is only one side of the story, no matter how much proof we believe we have to support our case. And we have to conscientiously seek to find out the other person's reality.

Therapist Mary Pipher talks about this in her book on dealing with aging parents, *Another Country*. She chose this title because she says that each generation really lives in a separate country in terms of worldview, beliefs, values, and behaviors. A lot of what she does in therapy is help middle-aged folks understand that their aging parents will always live in another country. That it's not meant as a personal insult, for instance, that they don't talk about how they feel, or say "I love you." It's a by-product of how they were raised.

Making an effort to understand relatives' behaviors, much like learning the customs of a foreign country, opens you up to compassion. Being connected and having that relationship is more important than who's right or who reaches out first. That awareness, along with some basic communication skills, can go a long way toward making the ties that bind more comfortable for us.

Of course, there will be times when tensions boil over. The goal of any argument is not victory, but progress and expansion. As I described in *Naomi's Breakthrough Guide,* in order to deal with our conflicts, we all sat down as a family one evening and agreed on some rules for communicating. I strongly suggest you do the same. Feel free to use ours as a jumping-off point:

## The Judd Family Feud Rules

1   No interrupting. (Wy used to say I'd make a great parole officer because I never let her finish her sentences.)

2   No shouting.

3   Everyone must realize we each have our own realities. (This is a big one for all family members to grasp.)

4   Everyone gets as much time as they need to fully express themselves.

5   Everyone should be prepared with their thoughts and solutions so time isn't wasted. This encourages the quiet, introverted ones to participate.

6   Pause to think before you speak so you address the person as if he or she is a friend.

7   No fair bringing others' opinions into it. (So-and-so said . . . )

8   Silence can be another form of arguing. Say what's on your mind.

9   Everyone needs to be aware that there will always be some "issue."

We came up with the powwow rules on our own in the early nineties. Since then, we've added many similar guidelines. After we saw how they really helped us, our family decided to also create a contract for the holidays so there'd be no more "holler/daze." Yes, Virginia, there is a Sanity Clause.

As blood relations, we assume (and remember: to assume makes an ass of u and me) that everybody thinks alike and wants the same things. Big mistake. Holidays are already intensely stressful. Period.

For Thanksgiving dinner 2005, all three households (husbands included) submitted a list what they wished for and what they didn't want. We faxed our lists to one another. Wishes included taking a group photo around the table; the oldest one says the grace; take a walk after the meal; everyone says what they are grateful for during dessert; etc. What we didn't want: talking showbiz, politics, or anything depressing, etc. After deciding on the menu and who was responsible for each dish, we figured out the assignments. Grace did place cards, Elijah filled water glasses, the guys were responsible for cleanup. We all were very pleased at how smoothly our day went. It was one of the best Thanksgivings we ever had!

It's important to put things in writing and give everyone a copy to keep so no one can claim he or she "forgot." All of us signed the contract. I even put it in the scrapbook where the family photo is in the front of my daytimer. This idea, to allow each member to express his or her wishes and concerns, worked so beautifully we plan to make it a habit before any major get-together.

Communicating well in stressful family situations is crucial. But equally important are healthy family relationships, says UCLA psychology professor Shelly Gable. For example, what would you say when a loved one comes or calls with good news? She offers four possible responses, only one of which helps improve the relationship. Here's what she means: Your son calls and says, "I've gotten a bonus and decided to use the money to build an addition on my house." How do you respond?

1   "That's great! Your boss must have realized what a fabulous job you are doing. Let's be sure to celebrate the next time you're here. What kind of addition are you thinking of?"

2   "That's nice, dear."

3   "That is so typical of you. You can't hold on to a dime. Always spending, spending, spending. You're going to end up in the poorhouse."

4   "When are you going to visit me?"

The first response is the one that helps create positive relationships. She calls it active constructive. You respond enthusiastically and positively to what is said, unlike number 4, in which you totally ignore what's said and go right to your own agenda. Number 2 sounds like you are disinterested, which doesn't help the person feel you are part of the event. The worst is number 3, when you don't respond positively at all but take the opportunity to give a lecture about the person's flaws and failings. That one actively destroys relationships.

## Goofy Grandma: Hip Hip Hooray

"[Having a grandchild] is like leasing a car, because you can turn it back in when the car misbehaves."
—JOHN LARROQUETTE

When I was in my early fifties, I entered the wonderful world of grandparenting. That's typical, say folks who study these things—most people become grandparents between forty-nine and fifty-three; by the time they are sixty-six, 75 percent of Americans have taken on this delightful new role.

As I've learned firsthand, it's a joyride. You get to be part of the growth and development of these miraculous beings, offer the wisdom you've learned from your own parenting, and see the world afresh again. And you don't have to deal with any of the drudgery parts—homework, cleaning rooms, making sure they eat their vegetables, etc. Mae West once said, "You're never too old to become younger," and grandkids sure help us do that. That's the best part. Grandchildren help us reconnect to our joy, to laugh and play. We may not be able to discover what it's like to swim in a creek for the first time again but we can revisit experiences through their eyes. (Did you see the email going around the internet about kids talking about love? One of my favorites was from Karl, age five: "Love is when a girl puts on perfume and a boy puts on shaving cologne and they go out and smell each other.")

Kids need their grandparents too. Research now shows that the brain is hardwired to connect to other people from birth. Through the connections with caring others, it develops its own potential. Parents can't do it all, even if they do it well. The brain needs connections to a variety of adults. We grandparents provide vital support. Through their relationship with us, grandchildren receive boosts to their self-esteem and have a greater chance to reach their potential. We can help them learn about their family history and customs and develop a positive attitude toward aging. They will understand they're linked in a long chain of belonging.

I keep a special drawer in my house full of gags and practical jokes that Grace and Elijah run to as soon as they come in the door—Groucho Marx glasses, whoopee cushions, masks, rubber chickens . . . you name it. I enjoy practical jokes as much as they do. And of course I always dress up at Halloween with them. Last year, Wy, Roach, Grace, Elijah, Larry, and I went trick-or-treating together.

Traditions are celebrations passed through the generations. It's one of our most important roles as grandparents to create or pass on rituals.

Ever thought of creating your own tradition? When my nephew Brian turned thirteen, we realized that Christians have no equivalent of a bar mitzvah. My other nephew and niece are Jewish and we'd enjoyed attending their bar and bat mitzvahs, so we came up with our own rite of passage to celebrate Brian's becoming a teen. The whole family got together for Brian's birthday, and after supper we formed a circle in the backyard. Brian's dad Mark laid a red robe on Brian's shoulders and ceremoniously announced, "May you be clothed in righteousness and God's protection." Mom Middy placed a crown upon his head and lovingly wished, "May you remember that your head and your heart should rule your life." Then Nana, his grandmother, lit a candle, approached him, and expressed her hopes for his future. As Mom finished, I took the flame from her candle for my turn. We continued in chronological order. We'll all remember how magical and unique the ceremony was. It will be repeated when Elijah and Grace come of age. I hope this story will spur ideas for you to come up with some rituals for your own family.

Even if you don't have grandchildren yourself, you don't have to miss out on all the fun and love in this role. You can become a "grandparent" to a niece's children or a neighbor's kids. Or become a foster grandparent. Foster grandparents serve as mentors, tutors, and caregivers for at-risk children and youth with special needs through a variety of community organizations, including schools, hospitals, orphanages and day-care centers. To learn more about the program, call 800-424-8867 or check the website at www.seniorcorps.gov.

Just like dealing with adult children, knowing the rules of the road helps prevent accidents. Here are mine:

1    Love your grandkids just for who they are, not for who you think they should be.

2    You are not the parent. Don't interfere with the parents' right to raise their child the way they see fit.

3    Check in with parents before giving extravagant gifts. Tiffany might want a pony but the family may not be able to handle it. You don't need to buy their love.

4    Avoid complaining, especially about their parents. Set an example by your positive behavior for the kind of adult you want them to become.

5    You have the right to express your boundaries and require good behavior when the grandkids are in your presence or home.

6    Babysit when you want, not because you feel guilty. Resentful care is not doing your grandchildren any favors.

7    Make seeing you a joy, not a burden. Remember—it's about fun!

# Caring for Those Who Cared for Us

"Getting old is not for sissies."
—JOHN P. GRIER

The other night I dreamed that I was back in my childhood home where my mother still lives. Mom had on her bathrobe, pajamas, and slippers, dangling rhinestone earrings, a big necklace, and a crown. The house was falling down and there were strange people there who were using her and her house.

When I awoke, I realized that the dream represented my concern because Mom lives alone and doesn't have much family in Ashland. As I get older, so does my mother. Like so many of us baby boomers, I'm now facing the reality that my parent could soon need ongoing support.

The dream made me realize that my siblings and I need to get together soon with and without Mom to have some straightforward conversations. We've got to decide what to do when Mom needs care. Right now, at seventy-nine, she's still able to take care of herself. Her house is everything to her—she's moved it twice and is still fixing it up. It's where we all grew up, a symbol of what the family once was. She just won't give up on that.

You too may be facing questions of what to do about an elderly relative. The answers aren't simple. Folks over eighty-five are the fastest-growing demographic in the country. Nearly forty-five million Americans, the vast majority women, are caring for adult family members. At a time when you thought things would be easier, you may instead be facing financial, emotional, and physical challenges as you struggle to care for a frail relative. You may need to learn the ins and outs of Medicare while trying to manage your parents' decision-making processes and deal with siblings who aren't helping. You may feel angry, guilty, or afraid of what's coming next. These feelings are all normal, but studies show that it is much easier to deal with the practical challenges than the emotional ones.

Research says that elders who live with their families fare better in thinking and ability to care for themselves than those in retirement homes. In most other cultures, children and extended family consider it not only their duty but also their pleasure to take care of the elderly. Worldwide, most people still live in a three-generational unit.

In America, more and more of us are putting our elderly in assisted living (if we can afford the high cost) because they are seen as a nuisance to our fast-paced lifestyle. But when we warehouse older people, their brains and bodies atrophy more quickly. For instance, regular contact with family reduces the risk of death from stroke and heart attack. We need to find ways to stay close to one another. That may mean moving Dad in with you, or moving nearer to him.

Recently, on the street in downtown Franklin, I chatted with ninety-year-old Rudell Martin, who told me, "I'm not really old because I still travel." She lives with her daughter who, as she puts it, "is absolutely wonderful. She treats me with every kindness in the world. We like to do things together. When I came to live with her, her husband was still alive and he was my buddy. We watched the ball games together. I recommend being ninety to everybody."

Terry Hargrave, professor of counseling at West Texas A&M, suggests that instead of just dumping responsibilities on one person, family members should get together, look at all the circumstances, and commission one person to be in charge. That person has the power to make decisions and to ask for help when needed. It helps, says Hargrave, to have the role acknowledged and supported by others. Then the rest of the family can give support and appreciation to the caregiver, looking out for when he or she needs a break, a bit of pampering, or time off.

There may be options other than family care. I support the concept of a project in India where widows and orphans are now living together in a community. The kids get grandmas to take care of them and the widows get much needed income and a reason to live. Some elders in the United States are now choosing to form intentional families made up of several generations and share housing.

Whatever your solution, adult children and their parents need to understand the kind of help that's truly beneficial. Longevity researchers have discovered, like Rudell Martin did, that the kind of help that people primarily need as they get older is emotional and social support, not physical help. That's because the more you do for older folks, the less they'll do for themselves and the faster they'll lose their capacity to be independent. We need to be there for loved ones emotionally, for companionship, but let them be independent as long as possible. Remember, at any age you best use it or lose it!

In this country, when you talk independence, the first thing that comes up is driving. As in, when and how to take away the car keys. Larry and I had to confront this with his dad. He drove a school bus and one day we realized he was not capable of doing it safely anymore. He was a gentle man who loved kids. And that's how we got to him. We told him it wasn't safe for the kids. It was very hard but typical of the sort of conversations that we have to be willing to have with our parents.

Of course, there are illnesses that don't allow for independence. Alzheimer's and other forms of senile dementia are particularly tragic. Ann and Nancy Wilson of the band Heart, visiting us at the farm, described their mom's decline with Alzheimer's as "like her personality was being erased." If a parent of yours is suffering from an all-consuming illness, my blessings on you—caregiving is the work of the soul. Please be realistic about what kind of help you can offer and still keep your own balance. Various options exist—care at home with help, adult day care, continuous care retirement communities. Don't forget the Family and Medical Leave Act, which allows qualified workers to take twelve weeks of unpaid leave in any twelve-month period to care for a family member, including a parent.

You don't have to have all the answers. How could you? None of us has journeyed down your particular road. Don't feel guilty about what you can't do. Factor in your own needs and ask for help.

When our friend Merlyn Littlefield's dad was in the latter stages of Alzheimer's, Larry invited him and his wife, Eileen, and several other friends our age over for supper. We pulled the lawn chairs together around him under the big tree in our backyard and sat there listening to Merlyn. It might have been the first time he really dealt with his father's disease. We all felt so bad for him but realized that just being there was what he needed from us. Merlyn eventually had to move his dad close by and put him in assisted living. It's very comforting knowing you don't have to face your difficulties alone.

Dealing with aging relatives can be a chance to have a new growth experience. It may require that we

- face our own fears about death

- pack up our emotional baggage from the past (or else we'll find ourselves in endless resentment—why am I helping this person who treated me so terribly when I was a child?)

- deal with other people's judgments about our choices

- set boundaries

- learn to say no without guilt if too many demands are placed on us

These are all things worth knowing how to do by the time you reach our age. Look at it this way, caring for our elderly parents may be the chance we've been needing to finally grow up ourselves. What a gift!

## Your Turn Now

- Have you had a meaningful moment with a family member this week? If not, why? One woman suggested that her father, her teenage daughters, and she write on the same four themes each month. At the end of each month, they would mail each other the writings. She then created four new themes. Topics included everything from favorite music to best holiday memories.

- Strong boundaries make happy families. Do you know what yours are? Not only in terms of what you will and won't put up with from relatives but also what you are willing to give or not? What are your money boundaries? Your respect boundaries? Your caretaking boundaries? Take time to decide before they are put to the test.

- What have you learned of value from your children? The Harvard Study of Adult Development discovered that folks who grow old successfully are more able to learn from the next generation.

- When someone in your family disappoints or angers you, can you let it go within a day? A week? The capacity to let go of grudges is one of the greatest family menders we have. If you have trouble letting go of past hurts, please read *Naomi's*

*Breakthrough Guide.* It can help you learn and heal from the past. Another great resource is: *I'm OK, You're My Parents: How to Overcome Guilt, Let Go of Anger, and Create a Relationship That Works* by Dale Atkins, PhD. You've seen Dr. Dale on my Hallmark Channel show as well as the *Today* show.

■ Sometimes we are so disconnected or estranged from children or grandchildren that all we can do is an affirmation like this one: *I love you and wish the best for you. Despite the difficulties we eventually will find our way back together.* These well wishes keep your heart open and may help build a bridge back to the other person. Perhaps you can find a way to even express it to them via a card or phone message.

■ Are there some courageous conversations you need to have with your parents? Questions such as: Do you have enough money? What if you get sick? Where will you live if you can't live by yourself? Do you have a will? If you are not sure what questions to ask, you might want to get the booklet *Caring Is Not Enough: The Most Important Questions You Can Ask.* It gives over seventy questions and is available for $8 at www.caringisnotenough.net. Before tackling your parents for a conversation, involve your siblings as much as possible so they don't feel you are going behind their back and your parents will know that you are all concerned. Decide who is going to discuss which issues. Don't do it over turkey dinner on Thanksgiving—pick a low-key situation. Talk about yourself first: "I just signed a durable power of attorney for health care. Have you?" Use examples from friends or other relatives: "Wasn't that awful that Lou's parents both had Alzheimer's? Do you have a plan if that happens to

Dad and you?" Experts say that it's easier for most people to talk first about health issues, then the money stuff. Let them know they are the boss but you are there to help. Understand if they are more comfortable talking to a professional rather than a family member. What's important is that they have a plan. Make sure you know who knows it.

- Are you caring for an elderly parent? Figure out ways not to do it by yourself. Call in your friends as resources, people who've gone through it already and have ideas. Join a support group. Or get support from the Family Caregiver Alliance (800-445-8106; www.caregiver.org) or Children of Aging Parents (800-227-7294; www.cars4caregivers.org). Or try Eldercare Locator (800-677-1116; www.eldercare.gov), which specializes in putting caregivers in touch with local resources that can help in your community. Also try www.alz.org/carefinder. It's sponsored by the Alzheimer's Association but is open to anyone looking for care for someone at home, an assisted living facility, or a nursing home. A great magazine is *Caring Today.* It has articles on everything from lotions for bedsores to preventing caregiver burnout. Also, be sure you make time for yourself—there's a thin line between devotion and martyrdom.

- Try viewing family members whom you find challenging as spiritual helpers. Instead of thinking, "Why are they this way?" ask yourself, "What lesson is this person helping me learn? How can I grow from this experience?" I've discovered that our elders and children are our greatest teachers.

"Of all the self-fulfilling prophecies in our culture, the assumption that aging means decline and poor health is probably the deadliest."
—MARILYN FERGUSON

# 8 | *As Good as It Gets:* Staying Fit in Mind and Body

SOMETHING INTERESTING HAPPENS when you identify and confront your greatest fear. I discovered mine when Wy and I were on the 1991 Farewell Tour. Our cop du jour—the police officer in that particular town riding on the bus as our security guard—and I were having a woman-to-woman talk. Because of my hep C, she wondered, "Are you afraid of dying?" After consideration, I replied, "No, because I believe in the hereafter." "Well, what are you most afraid of?" she probed. It was the first time I ever thought about it, but I realized my biggest fear is being dependent on others. Having been a nurse, I've seen way too many bedridden people of all ages. One of the reasons I became a nurse is I can't stand seeing people in pain or not being able to function as they wish. Being self-reliant my whole life, I highly value my ability to do it myself. Is independence a big part of who you are too? I want to be fully alive as long as I am living.

I'm now vigilant about taking good care of myself because hep C's threat to incapacitate was a major wake-up call. I decided to keep my body, mind, and spirit functioning well for absolutely as long as possible.

What's your greatest fear? Do you worry about someday becoming dependent? Do you associate getting older with becoming dependent? A desire to remain independent and alert, combined with my love of learning, fuels my studies in body/mind/spirit health. I've befriended many of the top scientists and holistic doctors in the world.

Keep on reading and I'll prove that aging is not necessarily going to lead to dependence. That's a misconception. Are you hip to the difference between chronological and biological age? Chronological is the age on your driver's license. It's how many years since your birth. Biological age refers to the age of your cells, which is determined not only by genes but also by lifestyle. That's right, all those choices you've been making. The National Institute on Aging announced that much of what we have thought of as symptoms of aging—aching joints; loss of flexibility, strength, and memory—are really due to disuse. Yes, disuse! A great example is Joseph Pilates, the father of the Pilates core strength exercise program. He had the biological body of a forty-year-old man when he died at the chronological age of eighty-six in a fire.

How fast our biological clock ticks has a lot to do with certain cells that are our brain's timekeepers. When they get whittled down to a certain length, they begin to shut off certain functions. These timekeepers, called telomeres, are influenced by diet, exercise, and whether you smoke, drink, or take drugs. Our daily lifestyle choices, therefore, influence when these timekeepers switch off. Yippee!

I'm sharing what works for me to give you some ideas, information, and direction. Be sure to consult a doctor you trust who can take your particular medical condition or symptoms into account when deciding on your best diet and exercise program.

# A Waist Is a Terrible Thing to Mind

"A man of sixty has spent twenty years in bed and over three years in eating."

—ARNOLD BENNETT

This is an important chapter because excess weight makes us look older and slows us down. Are you thick and tired of it? When it comes to eating right, remember Mom's advice: All things in moderation. For instance, Ashley came home from two months of being on a movie set and wanted a home-cooked meal. Fresh corn on the cob, green beans, new potatoes, fried chicken, and yes, apple pie. But this was a special occasion. The trick is not to eat such things every day. I do track the latest recommendations for a healthy diet and generally follow them.

Food is the medicine of our future. When you open your refrigerator, think of it as opening a medicine cabinet. Science is discovering that many of the diseases associated with aging have to do with inflammation in the body. It's important to choose a healthy diet that you can stick to daily and long term. My diet is one that has been shown to be anti-inflammatory, low in cholesterol, high in antioxidants (natural substances that help protect the body), and good for you whatever your age: lean protein (mostly from fish, chicken, or vegetables like soybeans), large quantities of fruits and vegetables (most Americans still don't eat enough), good fats such as those found in avocados, olive oil, and nuts (especially walnuts, which are rich in omega-3 fatty acids), which are good for preventing heart disease and stroke.

And eating whole grains. Nine out of ten Americans do not get the recommended amounts of whole grains or fiber. Soluble fiber found in vegetables, beans, and fruits removes toxins and slows absorption of carbohydrates and sugar into the bloodstream. Most of us eat less than a third of the fiber we should. We should be getting 30 grams a day.

Generally, I have red meat just a couple times a week. It has been linked to high cholesterol, heart attacks, colon cancer, and, recently, rheumatoid arthritis. Okinawans, those fabulously long-lived healthy folks who eat mostly fish and plant-based proteins, have 80 percent fewer heart attacks than North Americans. Try to eat fish several times a week, which turns out to be good for your brain too, particularly salmon, sardines, and mackerel. One study found that eating fish at least once a week can slow age-related mental decline by at least three to four years.

The movie *Super Size Me* stopped a lot of folks from going to drive-throughs and really made them conscious of their sugar and fat intake. I haven't had a dark soda in twenty-three years. Clear ones once in a while, but watch for artificial sweeteners in diet colas. Eating lots of fruits and veggies of different colors has been shown to give protection against age-related diseases such as cancer, cardiovascular disease, and neurodegenerative disease. Fresh berries, tomatoes, sweet potatoes, orange and yellow fruits, cabbage, broccoli, Brussels sprouts, and dark leafy greens like collards and chard contain antioxidants and are all great disease preventers.

Good carbs, healthy fats, and protein can be included at each meal, keeping in mind the recommendation that our calorie intake should come 45 to 65 percent from carbohydrates, 20 to 35 percent from fat, and 20 to 30 percent from protein.

My main meal of the day is usually lunch, which may include fish or chicken, fresh fruit, and veggies. I shy away from anything white—bread, pretzels, crackers, potatoes, pasta, etc. Dinner is sometimes leftovers from lunch. I try to have salads or veggies such as broccoli or asparagus every day.

Life span studies done at Harvard that tracked folks over fifty years found that alcohol has a great deal to do with aging poorly. Drinking more often creeps up on people as they get older. Drinking too much interferes with sleep, impairs memory, causes weight gain, endangers the liver, and impairs the body's ability to get the nutrition it needs. It also interferes with our relationships and causes isolation. Because our bodies have more fat and less muscle and water (because muscle is mostly water) than younger people, the concentration of alcohol in our bloodstream is greater. In case you don't know what amount is considered safe, it's 5 ounces of wine, 12 ounces of beer, or 1.5 ounces of 80-proof alcohol a day for women, twice that amount for men.

My daily beverage is low-carb cranberry juice mixed with seltzer. Raised on Pepsi, I want something with fizz and flavor so I feel like I'm getting a real beverage. I also like Crystal Light, especially the pink lemonade. To drink plenty of water, I add lots of lemons for flavor. (Here's a cooking tip. Put your limes and lemons in the microwave for forty seconds. It doubles the juices and increases the flavor because it releases the oils from the rind as well as the pulp.)

Do you get headaches? Are you aware that not drinking enough water facilitates them? Eight glasses of water a day keeps your body hydrated and helps all your chemical processes. Herbal teas, especially green and mate, contain good antioxidants. Pomegranate juice possesses strong antioxidant and anti-inflammatory properties. Studies show that plant chemicals in pomegranates inhibit cancer cell proliferation.

# Into the Waistland

"Middle age is when your age starts to show around your middle."
—BOB HOPE

The average American woman is 5'4" and 164 pounds. The average man is 5'10" and weighs 191. Let's face it—we all are going to pack on a few extra pounds as the decades clip by. We're probably going to go up a size once we get past forty. It's normal to weigh a bit more than when we were younger. If I start feeling bad about it, I remind myself that I'd rather be a role model than a supermodel.

Forty-eight percent of us weigh ourselves every day. The thing is not to live by the scale, because when you wake up in the morning, the first ten minutes set the tone for your mood for the day. It's like having a bad-hair day. Once a week you can check in on the scales. You need to declare an absolute weight that you will not go over. For me I can never go over 140. If I get to that point, that's when I know I need to cut back. I begin by reminding myself that at every moment I can change my life. Food is fuel to do my activities. Sometimes I have to remind myself to eat only when I'm hungry. I have more to think about than to live just to eat.

That's not to say it's easy. Our metabolism slows down 5 percent per decade from our forties onward, which means that pretty much all we can do besides exercise and eat the right kinds of foods is eat less. (Five percent doesn't sound like a lot, but if you used to eat 2,000 calories a day in your twenties, by the time you are sixty you need only 1,800; that's a *lot* less food per day.)

Even before *French Women Don't Get Fat* by Mireille Guiliano hit bookshelves, I liked the commonsense principle: Eat what you want, just tiny portions. Don't count calories and don't skip meals. When you skip, you set off your body's I'm-going-to-starve response, which makes you overeat later. Make sure the food you eat is what you want. That's why I don't go for the low-carb bars or food. And really savor your food by paying attention when you're eating. I don't usually watch TV or read because it's too easy to eat too much when you're not aware.

Eating is a visual experience too. I use small plates and enjoy a ritual with a nice place mat. I often have a bud vase filled with fresh flowers. I pause and recognize the sacredness of the gift from nature I am receiving. Then I indulge my senses—taste, smell, sight—and eat slowly to savor each bite. This helps me be satisfied without stuffing myself. I cut myself off when I start to feel slightly full. The Okinawans do the same—they eat only until they are 80 percent full. Did you know that we really don't feel full until twenty minutes after we stop eating? If we eat until we're full, we end up eating 20 percent too much every meal.

Can you believe we spend $33 billion a year on dieting? Obviously it's not working. Sixty-five percent of adults are overweight. It's an inner hunger they are trying to satisfy.

I don't do the diet thing like some people who sacrifice all week and then have a day when they just eat whatever they want. My system is everyday awareness of food as medicine and fuel. I keep dangerous "bingey" foods—popcorn and tortilla chips (my personal downfall) and other salty, crunchy things—out of the house so I won't be tempted. Rather than using willpower, which is hard to maintain over time, I set my life up so that it's easy to eat right all the time.

Because I crave crunchy foods, I'll turn to healthy munchables such as carrots, celery, or whole-grain cereal like Grape-Nuts to satisfy my urge to chew. I often keep a salad in the refrigerator so it's right there. I carry nuts like walnuts in my purse.

When I am trying to lose weight, I pick a small goal—mine right now is ten pounds. Weight-loss experts say that no matter how much you have to lose, it's best to do it gradually—one to two pounds a week. To lose one pound per week, you need to reduce 500 calories a day through a combination of eating less and exercising more. Consider your reward and visualize it all the time.

One tip is to think ahead. For instance, if I am going to a dinner with friends, I eat lighter the rest of the day. If Wy or Ashley is coming to our house, I sit down and eat right before they get here because I can get so excited when I'm around my family that I inhale food without even thinking.

Bob Greene, Oprah's weight-loss guru, says the number one trick is not to eat after 7 P.M. Some experts claim that all that food just lies there while you're sleeping, converting to fat. In fact, at night you don't take time to prepare good food. You snack on high-calorie, high-fat, high-sugar treats.

Another trick is to really load up on veggies with high water content. Studies have shown that if you begin a meal with vegetable soup, you fill up on good-for-you veggies and so eat less of the more fattening items. Various studies have shown that it is easiest to lose weight and keep it off with water-rich foods (you know, lettuce and cukes and apples and all those other foods packed with fiber and vitamins) because you can eat a lot and therefore not feel hungry.

I used to skip breakfast. Not anymore—since I saw studies showing that skipping a morning meal can actually cause us to gain weight. So I eat something small like yogurt or a fruit smoothie.

Really, you must decide that you do want to be independent as you age and that you need to be healthy. Then figure out the ways that work for you. Dolly Parton used to weigh twenty-five plus pounds more than now. After her weight loss, we were sharing a dressing room, and I said, "You're so little. Do you use Chap Stick for deodorant now?" When I asked her how she did it, she chirped, "Well, I eat six tiny meals a day." Many weight-loss experts are suggesting that. But if you're on the road, how can you do that? Thank goodness for salad bars.

Added weight brings with it many health hazards—increased risk for high blood pressure, high cholesterol, diabetes, heart attack, stroke, the list goes on and on. Overeating has now usurped smoking as the most preventable disease-causing behavior. It leads to a shorter, less healthy life. Studies of people who make it to a hundred find that few have ever been obese (which may account also for their lower cancer rates).

If grateful aging is really about being the best you can be, no matter what age, you're not being your best if you're carrying a lot of extra weight. To maintain our dignity as we age, we must not let ourselves go.

For some, like Wynonna, losing weight is a deep source of pain and struggle. I'm trying to do whatever I can to help her on this front. That's why I was willing to go on *Oprah* with her and Ashley and my mom, her nana, to support her. Oprah has been very honest about her own challenges with overeating. She tried many things but ultimately realized that "Getting my lifelong weight struggle under control has come from a process of treating myself as well as I treat others in every way." I truly believe you've got to love the person in the mirror. In other words, to lose weight you must cultivate healthy self-esteem. *Fat Is a Family Affair* is a great book. All addictions are a no-fault disease. All addictions are about trying to ease the pain of living.

After Wynonna was on *Oprah,* Oprah asked me, "What did you think when you saw Wy on our show from your home?" My immediate response was how I was struck by what an unusual celebrity she is. So many female singers are rail thin and are famous for perfect images and perfect bodies but have little talent or value to offer. But here is Wynonna, who is enormously talented and immensely likable because she was willing to admit, "I'm scared. I've made bad, bad choices. I'm asking for help because I want to change." Do you see yourself in Wy?

I trust that Wy will find her way. As her mother, I can give her unconditional love, sincere encouragement, and space.

# The Scoop on Supplements

"A vitamin is a substance that makes you ill if you don't eat it."
—BIOCHEMIST ALBERT SZENT-GYORGYI,
NOBEL PRIZE FOR MEDICINE, 1937

I'm a fan of vitamin supplementation since we get only about a third of the nutrients we need on our fork. And to figure out which to take, I trust the recommendations by my dear friend Dr. Andrew Weil. Andy is a medical doctor who has devoted the past thirty years to developing, practicing, and teaching others about the principles of preventative and integrative medicine.

In his comprehensive book *Healthy Aging,* he shares his recommendations for supplements based on the latest research from around the world. For more information on his supplement and dietary recommendations, as well as his ideas for meal planning and recipes, check out www.healthyaging.com. Here are some of his recommendations.

## Vitamins and Minerals

- Four antioxidants to help prevent cancer, heart disease, and other chronic illnesses: vitamin C, 200 milligrams a day; vitamin E, 400 IU of natural mixed tocopherols (d-alpha tocopherol with other tocopherols, or, better, 80 milligrams of natural mixed tocopherols and tocotrienols); selenium, 200 micrograms of an organic (yeast-bound) form; mixed carotenoids, 10,000–15,000 IU daily.

- A daily multivitamin/multimineral that provides at least 400 micrograms of folic acid (helps prevent heart attack, stroke, cancer, and osteoporosis, as well as memory depression in older adults) and at least 1,000 IU of vitamin D (helps with the absorption of calcium). It should contain no iron and no preformed vitamin A (retinol).

- Supplemental calcium, preferably as calcium citrate. Women need 1,200–1,500 milligrams a day, depending on dietary intake of this mineral; men should get no more than 1,200 milligrams of calcium a day from all sources.

## Other Dietary Supplements

- If you are not eating oily fish at least twice a week, take supplemental fish oil, in capsule or liquid form, 1–2 grams a day. Fish oil contains omega-3 fatty acids, which can lower triglycerides, increase good HDL cholesterol, help minimize inflammation and blood clotting, and keep blood vessels healthy. Look for molecularly distilled products certified to be free of heavy metals and other contaminants. Cook with olive oil, try steaming or sautéing or stir-frying.

- Talk to your doctor about going on low-dose aspirin therapy, one or two baby aspirins a day (81 or 162 milligrams). As of 2006, it's been shown to reduce the risk of heart attack and stroke as well as reduce the risk of colon and prostate cancer.

- If you are not regularly eating ginger and turmeric, consider taking these in supplemental form. Concentrated extracts of these can help protect the body from common toxins.

- Add Co-Q10 to your daily regimen: 60–100 milligrams of a softgel form taken with your largest meal. I take it because I'm on a statin for high cholesterol. Co-Q10 may help prevent heart disease and Parkinson's as well as many other chronic diseases.

- If you are prone to metabolic syndrome (a combination of obesity, high blood pressure, and high blood sugar that raises the risk of heart disease), take alpha-lipoic acid, 100–400 milligrams a day.

## Pumping Iron

"A bear, however hard he tries, grows tubby without exercise."
— *POOH'S LITTLE INSTRUCTION BOOK*

Joke: "At my age the only reason I'd start exercising is so that I could hear heavy breathing again." If that sounds like you, it's time to get on the exercise bandwagon. It's good for your health, brain, spirits, and obviously your waistline. It's even more crucial as we age. It keeps you from losing too much muscle mass, keeps you flexible, gives you more energy, and maintains your sense of balance (which otherwise is often a casualty of aging; that's why so many folks over sixty-five fall). Between thirty-five and seventy, you lose 50 percent of your strength and 75 percent of your power, unless you keep working on it. A seventy-five-year-old man can look forward to an additional eleven years if he maintains a fitness routine, and women can gain thirteen more.

Many studies also show that exercise improves thinking ability in folks sixty to seventy-five as well as reduces stress and anxiety. It also slows aging—a fit body, says Walter M. Bortz II, MD, of Stanford University Medical School, grows old at the rate of $1/_2$ percent per year, while an unfit one deteriorates at 2 percent per year. (It may not seem like a lot, but multiply that by ten or twenty years and there's a big difference.) And once we get to a certain age, even those of us who've stayed thin without breaking a sweat have trouble keeping off the extra pounds without vigorous exercise. Movement increases circulation to remove toxins that promote aging. Exercise helps us maintain our appearance and therefore our self-confidence.

Dr. Pamela Peeke, a physician, nutritionist, stress reduction expert, and author, recommends that after the age of forty, we do at least forty-five minutes a day of some aerobic activity at least five to six days a week. In addition, at least thirty minutes twice a week of strength training and stretching (like yoga). Aerobic activity includes walking, swimming, biking, hiking, skiing, dancing, jumping rope, kickboxing, tennis, and rowing. Strength training can be lifting weights—either barbells or on machines like Nautilus—and circuit training.

Until recently, I'd never been to a gym or had a personal trainer. Since I fly several times a month, I walk through terminals instead of taking the moving sidewalk and take the stairs instead of the escalator. I say that the best exercise is one that you will really do!

But I noticed that my regular routine wasn't doing anything to take off the ten extra pounds that crept on after age fifty. Plus I've been learning about the necessity of resistance training to guard against loss of muscle tissue. Do you know that if you don't do strength training, you lose seven pounds of muscle or more every ten years? So I'm currently using a personal trainer to help me get going. Since I advocate mind, body, and spirit health, I'm feeling mentally relieved now that I'm finally doing it because it's been this nagging thing.

That gorgeous hunk you may have spotted on *Oprah* as Wy's trainer is Dominick Divito. A longtime family friend, a professional trainer, and a sixth-degree black belt, Nick now motivates me to exercise, plus he teaches me self-defense. Even if you're a small-framed female like me, Nick will help you understand that, again, prevention and awareness are our power. He shows us that our minds are our best weapon and he demonstrates how to react and make the right decisions when you are in a panicked state. Check out Dominick's book on personal safety, *Fight Back,* and his website, www.dominickdivito.com.

I was motivated to begin exercising when it clearly dawned on me that it can help me avoid illness, soreness, weakness, decreased sexuality, weight gain, etc. With health-care costs soaring, if you don't exercise now, pay attention now, you could end up in financial ruin. Exercise and pay attention now or literally pay later.

I plan to explore yoga next. It can help you lose or keep off weight. Studies have found that folks who do yoga tend to weigh less than those who don't. Yoga also aids in the proper functioning of the organs, nerves, and glands. It improves circulation and respiration—essential to cardiovascular fitness. It also improves digestion and coordination, and strengthens the immune system. Here's what Ashley says about it: "Yoga lets me be me, comfortable and open. If I have a scene in which I'm really uptight, or if I'm anxious, I like to open myself up. If you give it a chance, it will grow within you."

I was in a hotel preparing for a speech on women's health issues when a note was slipped under my door: "We know you're a Christian, so we hope you won't promote yoga in your presentation today." Many are misinformed, like this writer. Yoga isn't a religion. It's a method to create union of spirit, mind, and body. It's a discipline of movement taught even at the Young Women's Christian Association.

Another enjoyable form of movement for your whole life is tai chi. It's an ancient series of slow movements designed to create greater strength, balance, and peace of mind. Elderly Asian women have fewer falls because tai chi greatly enhances their sense of balance. But along with these milder forms of exercise you need to do vigorous exercise for cardio and other benefits.

So you know what you should be doing. But how to actually do it? You're interested because you're reading this. If your budget allows, a trainer is fabulous because he or she is there at a scheduled time to motivate you, to make sure you stick to it, to help you know how and when to push yourself. Many clubs have trainers that are not too expensive. If that's not an option, consider a circuit-training place like Curves, 21 Minute Convenience Fitness, or Ladies Workout Express. You follow a set routine in a set amount of time so it's harder to cheat.

Find an exercise buddy—the two of you can motivate and support one another. Every time I'm in the mall, I see mall walkers taking advantage of the stimulating sights, safety, and climate controlled indoors. Talk on the cell phone while you walk if it will help you get started. Get a dog so you'll have to walk. If you can't find thirty minutes at once, do ten minutes three times a day—a brisk miniwalk, for instance. Some studies have found that works even better, perhaps because it keeps metabolism high all day.

What also works for me is to think of exercise as a regimen like brushing your teeth, combing your hair, or bathing. You don't think about whether you're going to do it, you just do it for your body. It's automatic. I schedule exercise in my day planner so I do it no matter what. If you are traveling or if the gym is closed, or you're sitting by your mother's bedside in the hospital, take a walk. Whatever amount of time you've committed to, you do it no matter who or what else is pulling on you for attention. It's not an option any longer. It's become a matter of putting your own health on your radar screen. And when you fall off the wagon, and don't do it for a day or a week or a month, regroup and begin again.

Give yourself rewards along the way—a new sweater if you stick to it for a month, a massage. Not having the time is no excuse. While Wy and I were performing at the White House, I asked Condoleezza Rice what she does to deal with the unreal stress of being secretary of state. She responded, "Exercise." If she can do it with her schedule, we can!

## Both Are Better (Modern Medicine and Complementary Medicine)

"We delight in the beauty of the butterfly, but rarely admit the changes it has gone through to achieve that beauty."
—MAYA ANGELOU

As we age, finding the right doctor is even more crucial because our potential for disease goes up. Plus since we're living longer, you want someone who will not only be up on the latest treatments but also have the best preventive measures.

I am a great believer in integrated medicine because it combines the very best of the latest Western medicine with tried-and-true ancient techniques that are used in 85 percent of the world: techniques such as acupuncture, massage, meditation, biofeedback, chiropractic, aromatherapy, yoga, guided imagery, and supplements. Fortunately, more and more M.D.s are using the power of all these methods to achieve wellness.

Shop around for the right doctor. A website that might be useful is www.webmd.com. A good book on this topic is *You: The Smart Patient.* Get recommendations from friends, relatives, and other health-care professionals. Ask lots of questions and find out if she solves every problem with a pill or is well versed in all possible methods. Will he talk to you outside office hours if you have a question? Does she seem to genuinely care about you? Listen to you without interrupting? Is he covered under your medical insurance? What about the hospital that she is affiliated with? Do you feel comfortable in the office? Once you've got a good doctor, be sure to raise the medical issues that accompany aging.

Osteoporosis is a disease of aging in which your bones get brittle and porous, break easily, and don't heal well. Osteoporosis is responsible for more than 1.5 million hip, vertebrae, and other fractures every year. Four times as many of us gals get it as men, and the risk starts relatively young. Postmenopausal women are particularly at risk—we can lose up to 30 percent of the bone mass in our spines in just the first five years after menopause. Caucasian, small-framed women are more at risk.

So what can we do about it? It's never too late to have better bone health because no matter how thin our bones are now, we can reduce further bone loss and even conserve what we do have. My own sports medicine specialist, Dr. Tom Bartsokas, advises that first you get a bone density scan to see where you are and establish a baseline. Then make sure to take 1,500 mg of calcium every day, half in the morning and half at night. Calcium does more than keep our bones strong—it also helps keep us from getting fat, reduces cholesterol, may reduce colon cancer risk, and may protect against stroke. Dr. Tom also says vitamin $D_3$ deficiency among older folks has become epidemic in the United States. He recommends 1,200 IU daily. You can get it over the counter. Note: Your body will not absorb calcium without vitamin D$_3$. I try to get calcium–vitamin D$_3$ with every meal. Don't drink carbonated beverages with the calcium, as the phosphoric acid will leach the calcium from the bone.

Next, be sure to do weight-bearing exercise every day: walking, dancing, circuit training. Any exercise where you are carrying (yourself) or lifting weights. Third, don't smoke—it adds ten years to your bones besides all the other bad things it does to your lungs—and drink alcohol only in moderation (it inhibits the growth of new bone cells).

## To Replace or Not to Replace . . . That Is the Question

One of the most controversial and pressing issues about midlife is menopause. Women of all generations may lack access to scientific journals and time to equip themselves with this turning point in womanhood. Currently negative images, misconceptions, and half knowledge about menopause are causing unnecessary trepidation. It's hard to keep up with the latest medical research.

Some women are unabashedly and unapologetically menopausal. Former Manhattan gynecologist Dr. Patricia Allen formed an organization called Women's Voices for Change to spread the word that menopausal transition is actually a wonderful time of life. It's an opportunity for us to reevaluate ourselves, and you'll find out you're smarter, richer, and, yes, sexier than you were allowing yourself to be.

Dr. Allen's prescription is to remain aware of your choices. Just as we needn't take in more calories than we burn, we need to know we have the choice to be elegant, beautiful, well dressed, witty, and sexier in our later years. She insists, "One of the great lies is women over forty-five want to be younger. But we'd rather have a gun to our heads than to go back to our younger selves." Look out, she's out of estrogen and she's got a gun.

None of us knows what our midlife point is, since we can't know for certain how long we'll live. But we do know that females are born with all the equipment and eggs (ova) we'll ever have. It's simple math figuring when a woman starts menopause. Also, you can ask your mom and aunts at what point they became menopausal. If a girl starts her periods, menarche, around thirteen and ovulates once a month, at age fifty, she's pretty close to out of eggs. When I hit fifty, I informed Larry one morning over coffee, "Honey, I'm out of eggs." "That's okay," he responded dryly. "I'll have cereal."

For my hormonal health since I became menopausal at age fifty, I've worked closely with Dr. Joel Hargrove of Vanderbilt University in Nashville, one of the experts on bioidentical HRT. *Bio* refers to life, *identical* means the hormone replacement therapy uses molecules most like our own natural female hormones. He began his medical practice thirty-some years ago as a gynecologist specializing in working with women suffering with PMS. Fortunately for all of us, since he's followed his patients for thirty-plus years into their menopausal and post-menopausal phases, Dr. Hargrove is now very knowledgeable and specialized. And he knew for years that Premarin (made from the urine of pregnant mares, usually under questionable circumstances), Provera (synthetic progesterone), and Prempro (Premarin and progesterone in one pill) are not good for women's bodies. This is documented in many scientific reports. So Dr. Hargrove's research was validated when these widely prescribed treatments were discouraged by the Women's Health Initiative in 2002. The study, which included women fifty through seventy-nine, exposed a variety of health problems related to synthetic hormone replacement. Dr. Hargrove knows that the prescription bioidentical forms of replacement estrogen, progesterone, and testosterone are definitely better. Unfortunately, because these bioidenticals have not been studied, most misinformed conventional doctors may still think all HRT should be avoided. They're throwing the baby out with the bathwater. And women suffer.

Here's Dr. Hargrove's expert advice: "The three major sex hormones are estradiol, progesterone, and testosterone. They are present in all animals and both sexes, male and female. At menopause, they are dramatically reduced, which often results in a variety of symptoms that impact quality of life, including insomnia, hot flashes, diminishment of sexual desire and pleasure, brain activity, and memory.

"Many people will argue that menopause is a natural phenomenon, so taking hormones is unwarranted. Life expectancy was once a mere forty-seven years, and menopause, as today, occurred around fifty. Consider, however, women today can expect to live into their eighties. This means women today are spending an increasing period of their lives in a less-than-optimal hormone environment. That's why I suggest bioidentical hormone replacement therapy."

Dr. Hargrove finds that "if hormone replacement is elected, it is very important that nature is mimicked in as much detail as possible. And that's where bioidentical comes in. The same types of molecules are created in bioidentical hormones that were produced by your body. Since 1995, I have carefully chosen the transdermal application [meaning through the skin] of compounded lotions containing estradiol, progesterone and testosterone. Each individual has her own absorption pattern that must be predetermined by measuring blood levels for all three hormones. Once the level of hormones in the body is known and a pattern of absorption is established, it rarely changes with time. One of the reasons for avoiding taking HRT orally is that bioidentical transdermal administration lowers chances for blood clots and higher blood pressure. It also bypasses the liver. Estrogen and progesterone supplements at health food stores are unregulated and unpredictable."

I wholeheartedly agree with Dr. Hargrove that unless prior medical history contraindicates, women need to replace the estrogen, progesterone, and testosterone that their bodies stop producing at menopause. Hey, if your pancreas doesn't manufacture insulin, you need to supply it. If your thyroid stopped producing the hormone thyroxin, you take thyroid replacement for life.

As for the guys at midlife, women make 70 percent of health care choices for the family. So it's often up to us to schedule medical exams for spouses. Prostate cancer is the second leading cause of death for American men. Yet the blood test, PSA, is simple. Men treat their cars like women treat their bodies.

On the subject of medical tests, don't forget screening for colon cancer. Colorectal cancer, which is detectable with early screening, claims the lives of 56,000 Americans each year. By the time you hit fifty, you are at risk, so screening is absolutely necessary. Katie Couric, who lost her husband, Jay, to colon cancer, advises we take our doc's advice of how often to get tested.

I use my birth month, January, to celebrate my health and be grateful. That's when I get all my annual checkups from head to toe—eyes checked, teeth cleaned, mammogram, Pap smear, blood tests for cholesterol and cardiac fitness, and bone density. If I have any little spider veins (broken capillaries) on my legs, I even get sclerotherapy to get rid of them. (This procedure isn't covered by insurance.) Doing it all at once means I don't have to worry about my health for a whole year. And remember, an eye exam is just as important as the other tests. By age sixty-five, one in three Americans has some kind of vision-limiting disease. At sixty, I had cataract surgery. And not being able to see well has been linked to decline in brain function. Many eye diseases are treatable, so be sure to take good care of your sight.

# Yearning for Learning

"Old minds are like old horses: you must exercise them if you wish to keep them in working order."
—JOHN ADAMS

For those of us who worry about memory loss and fear Alzheimer's disease, there is great news from medical science. Many neuroscientists now believe the brain is capable of excellent performance into our hundreds and that aging by itself does not lead to dementia or Alzheimer's. Now that's worth remembering!

It was once believed that we are born with all the brain cells we were ever going to have and that we steadily lose them over time. But recently scientists have discovered that adults do generate new brain cells (neurons) and that we can grow new dendrites (the parts of our neurons that allow the cells to communicate with one another) to compensate for ones we've lost.

And we must make new connections. We need what scientists call cognitive reserve, meaning as much wiring as possible so that the loss of some old wiring won't turn all your lights off. The brain is a very complicated network of connections. The more connections, the less any loss matters. The way we create cognitive reserve is through lifelong learning. Here's the way I think of it—your brain constantly needs to be learning something or else it shuts down. Again, use it or lose it.

There's a correlation between less education and a higher rate of

Alzheimer's. Education definitely stimulates growth of neurons. That's why scientists who've studied folks who lived to a hundred recommend doing things that challenge us: crossword puzzles, writing poetry or keeping a journal, learning a new language or complicated dance such as the hula, or playing an instrument at least half an hour two to three times a week. Like physical fitness, the more intense and exertive it is, the better off our brains are. Like our muscles, our brains need to *work* to stay healthy (which is why big TV watchers tend to lose their mental capacity faster than those who use their brains).

Because of my medical background, I love the combination of medical science, psychology, and unsolved crime on forensic TV. It's like putting together a puzzle. Who, what, when, and why? I also attend mind/body/spirit conventions and read on the subject. Learning is like oxygen to me. Essential to life.

That's why I was fascinated to learn that, while we are all afraid of becoming forgetful, what is really happening is that we're not learning things as well in the first place, as Lawrence Katz, a professor of neurobiology at Duke University Medical Center, discovered. We need to do more for our mental fitness than crossword puzzles. The more we form associations using all of our senses—sight, sound, smell, taste, touch—the stronger our mental networks will be. Then remembering is easier. The reason we become forgetful in our forties and beyond is that we've created only one connection—say, a name to a face. When our brains are young, that's enough. But as we get older, we've met so many people that just the visual link isn't strong enough to call up the person. Come to your senses and use them.

It's not just about recall. Dr. Katz says we get into mental ruts that are deadening our brains if we're not forming new associations. So he invented something he calls neurobics. They are ways to develop strong connections throughout the brain. These are simple things you can do in your daily life to break mental routines and therefore create new pathways and strengthen your memory—things like taking a shower with your eyes closed so that you must rely on your other senses, putting the phone to your nondominant ear, unlocking your front door with your eyes closed, or brushing your teeth with your nondominant hand (including putting on and off the top to the toothpaste tube). You don't have to be a dental hy-genius to do it, either.

In a weird way, doing a good job brushing your teeth has something else to do with brain health. It turns out that gum disease in early life is more of an indicator of dementia than genes. Scientists are not sure why, but they think it may have something to do with an increase in inflammation, which is harmful to the brain as well as the body. How do you know when it's time to go to the dentist? When it's tooth hurty.

Of course trying new things will feel awkward, but that's the point. I will if you will. Any routine is brain-deadening because it requires a minimum of brain exercise. We need to create new pathways, and that means engaging as many of our senses as possible in something new.

People who drink vegetable or fruit juice at least three times a week may be less likely to get Alzheimer's than those who don't. Again, they don't know why but think it's because of polyphenols, which may protect the brain. Adding a glass of juice a day is a no-brainer!

A study in Holland found that taking 800 micrograms of folic acid a day boosts memory function. Older folks who did did as well on memory tests as though they were five and a half years younger. And take those supplements Dr. Weil recommended—the healthy older Okinawans I spoke of in earlier chapters have much lower incidents of Alzheimer's and other forms of senility. The reason? Their diet is high in vitamin E, which seems to help the brain. Vitamins C and B$_3$—niacin— also seem to help prevent brain deterioration.

Physical exercise is good for the brain too because it oxygenates the cells, increases blood flow to the brain, and releases those feel-good hormones. Exercise even increases IQ—up 7.5 percent in one study. And if you want even more of a brain boost, work out to music. Studies show that verbal ability went up in those who exercised to music, as opposed to those who exercised in silence.

It's estimated that five million Americans over sixty-five suffer from serious depression. The really depressing part is that a sizable percentage of them aren't getting treatment! Antidepressant medication, in combination with therapy, can help greatly. Treatment will also help prevent further illness and curb suicide.

Contrary to the long-held belief that our brain power inevitably declines as we age, Gene D. Cohen, MD, PhD, in his book *The Mature Mind,* argues that there are actually positive changes taking place in our minds. This renowned gerontologist and psychiatrist offers scientific research supporting the idea that our minds continue to grow in the second half of our lives. I was greatly encouraged by his findings that the brain's information-processing center achieves its peak density and reach between the ages of sixty and eighty.

My gal pal Dr. Mona Lisa Schulz tells me how our brain remodels itself and has enormous plasticity. New brain cells lead to new potential. Dr. Schulz's latest book, *The New Feminine Brain,* is chock-full of brain food.

## *Your Turn Now*

- Do you eat right and exercise enough? If not, what needs to change in your day so that you can? Are you willing to commit to those changes? What kind of help do you need to stick to it? Visualize the rewards.

- If you need to make a lot of changes, do it gradually. Make a 10 percent change—exercise 10 percent more, eat 10 percent more fruits and veggies, increase your fiber by 10 percent, eat 10 percent less. Each of these is so easy you will barely notice and you can make these changes one per month until you're doing them all. Then see if you can do another 10 percent, and so on.

- If fish is not your fave, commit to eating it on Fridays, the way Catholics used to. The day doesn't really matter. But studies show that eating it even once a week has real benefits for your arteries, heart, and brain.

- If weight is a real issue for you, consider getting help—from Overeaters Anonymous, therapy, Fat Is a Family Affair, or Geneen Roth's great books on emotional eating including *When Food Is Love.* You deserve a body that makes you feel good about yourself.

- Follow my suggestion and book your annual physical exam in your birthday month. Be sure to schedule every test you need. Maybe schedule lunch with a friend before the appointment.

- What do you do on a daily basis that helps your brain stay active? You might be interested in reading Lawrence C. Katz's book *Keep Your Brain Alive.* It's filled with creative suggestions for breaking out of mental ruts and exercising your brain.

- Add one new, mentally stimulating activity into your life. Take a writing workshop, join a book group, or take an adult ed course. Learn one new vocabulary word a week. If there's a college nearby, go to a lecture.

- To keep your mathematical ability, balance your checkbook without using a calculator. Then double-check your results. To strengthen your memory, don't rely on speed dial; memorize family's and friends' phone numbers.

- Say this affirmation: *I am healthy and strong. I am beloved of spirit and my body is the manifestation of spirit. I exhale all that is not useful to me. I inhale strength and vitality.*

"We can tell our values by looking at our check-book stubs."
—GLORIA STEINEM

# 9 | *Million Dollar Baby:* Looking as Good as You Feel

LET'S SEE: Botox or anthrax? Last year Americans spent as much on anti-aging products and procedures as Homeland Security. That's an indication of how lucrative the skin trade is and that our vanity is at least as important to us as our safety. (By the way, I've never used Botox 'cause I need the option of raising my eyebrow to shoot Wy and Ashley "the look.")

As we age, it's easy to neglect the physical aspect of our being, to let ourselves go. But it's important for our inner happiness not to. Because the way you face yourself in the mirror is the way you face your life. Looking good on the outside helps boost self-esteem and confidence on the inside. When you feel confident, you're more comfortable handling what life dishes out. It also boosts your awareness of your well-being and helps you make choices to have a better life. Healthy self-esteem also motivates us to take note and take care of our emotional centers.

We just feel more worthy and start attracting better people and circumstances.

Your breakthrough starts with realizing that the answer is not found in makeup or cosmetic surgery. It's about self-acceptance, loving yourself, and then taking inventory of your life. Whether it's putting on makeup or putting on airs, many women wear masks. (Did you hear what happened when Tammy Faye removed all her makeup? They found Jimmy Hoffa.)

Be careful of the mask you choose. The French writer Alfred de Musset said, "For it reveals you more than it hides you." I'm here to give you permission to refuse to allow others to define who or what you are. (Mary Kay Ash, founder of the very successful cosmetics company, once quipped, "So many women just don't know how great they really are. They come to us all vogue on the outside and vague on the inside.")

My bathroom has a big mirror. I go there to "reflect" sometimes. The beginning of each day and the closing of each night are opportunities for not only your beauty routine but also to get in touch with your inner self, the deeper you. How about acknowledging how unique and special you are instead of simply looking at your superficial reflection, checking for flaws? These are moments to get in touch with those unexpressed parts of yourself. It is a time for you to acknowledge that you are already all you need to be. That you can be anything you want and do whatever you choose. You are worthy. You do deserve the best! Remember, how you face yourself is how you face others.

Looking your best doesn't have to be costly or time-consuming. You can make your home your spa and your bathroom your sanctuary. You can do all your beauty treatments yourself. I do. I don't do professional manicures or pedicures. I keep nail polish remover and clippers in the glovebox of my car because I do my nails in the car while Larry drives. As for facials, I've had only one my entire life. It's a waste of money to pay someone to give you a facial, when, with the right products, you can do it yourself. So money should not be a hindrance to looking great.

If my mom had Halo shampoo, Sweetheart soap, Jergens hand lotion, and a tube of lipstick, she was good to go. That practicality was born out of having four kids and a husband who worked at a gas station and came home in greasy overalls. My mother has never had anything "done." Forget face-lift—no collagen, no Botox. She did have a facial once, actually. Wy and I were performing in Las Vegas and I wanted her to go home to Ashland, Kentucky, and tell Aunt Roberta and Martha Compton and her best friends all about it. My grandmother, Sally Ellen Judd, my dad's mom, was a farmer's wife, unconcerned about her looks and too busy living. All of these women helped me learn that what mattered most was being defined from within.

The body is the home of the soul. I firmly believe that we're not only supposed to age *gratefully* but also *great*-fully—and that means looking wonderful.

"You can be gorgeous at twenty, charming at forty, and irresistible for the rest of your life."
—COCO CHANEL

## Full Esteem Ahead

"I'm tired of all this nonsense about beauty being only skin-deep. That's deep enough. What do you want, an adorable pancreas?"
—JEAN KERR

When you're a celebrity, every makeup line, hair-care line, and skin-care line sends you its products. Plus when I'm in a different city and using a local hairdresser or makeup artist, they bring me their favorite salon brand products. For over twenty years, I've sampled everything out there in the beauty field. When I didn't have money, I got squirts of the sample perfumes at the drugstore before dates because I couldn't afford to buy it. Later, when I was able to buy a $50 jar of moisturizer or $150 cream in an expensive store that promised the moon, I was never satisfied. Either it was overpriced or didn't fulfill its promise. I felt like a sucker.

I became interested in the skin and skin-care formulas while studying for my nursing degree. I began making my own soap back in Kentucky over twenty-five years ago. I even put a patent on Naomi's Homemade Soap in the seventies. When folks asked me what I was going to do when I quit singing, I'd jokingly reply that I planned to turn my garage into a beauty shop.

I've always wanted to know what's inside every beauty product. I am also aware of the importance of healthy ingredients, but I'm outraged at how overpriced they are. Ninety percent of the cost of the products is for packaging and marketing. So when my own dermatologist, who helped create many skin-care lines, asked me to start a skin-care line, I was game.

I was inspired by an incident at the Ivy restaurant in L.A., my favorite restaurant in the world. Five or six women were drinking margaritas, laughing and carrying on at the next table. I was just enjoying the residual vibe from their girls' night out. When they recognized me, they identified themselves and wanted to know my skin-care secrets. (I am blessed to have inherited porcelain skin from my redheaded mama, but there's more to it than that.)

Sort of embarrassed, I replied, "I'm a happy person, and happiness is the best cosmetic." But people have asked me about my skin-care secrets my whole adult life, so I thought it was time to state my age and share my regimen. In my public image as a singer, a celebrity, and the mother of two famous daughters. I've come to know more than you can imagine about skin care, beauty tips, hair, makeup, and fashion. It dawned on me I have something truly useful to share. Not only about how to go about looking good, but more important, how looking good and feeling good are related. Pretty soon my Esteem Skincare Line was born.

Once I began to encourage women to take practical steps to look better, to take care of themselves in general, I realized they began demanding more out of their existence. They tell me their stories wherever I go. One woman who entered the clinical trials for Esteem told me she hadn't been feeling good about herself for some time. As she began to pay more attention to her looks, she had a transformation. She was even able to lose the fifteen pounds she'd been struggling with for years. Another woman in the trials soon noticed as she was taking better care of herself, her daughter began holding herself in higher regard. She was setting a good example for her.

Once when I told an older woman how pretty she was, she corrected me, saying, "I am beautiful, not pretty. Pretty is on the outside. Beautiful is inside. If I feel beautiful inside, then that's the way I look outside." Amen, sister.

I deal with the biological issues of aging skin that every woman has, but I have additional skin needs because I'm in so many weather extremes. I'm in steamy Hawaii one day, dry Las Vegas the next, and then frosty New England. I'm also on airplanes a lot, which is like being in the Sahara as far as your skin is concerned. When you're under the spotlight, whether it's in a TV studio or a photo session and certainly on stage, it's like "take your face and bake at 350 degrees for two hours." I *have* to have great cleansers and moisturizers.

For my skin-care line, I demanded the freshest ingredients and of course no animal testing. Products had to be potent, indulge all the senses, be simple and easy to use, and be economical.

With my dry, sensitive mature skin, I was the guinea pig for testing my own products.

I've very proud of the results. We also utilize aromatherapy, so that it's really not only the best biomedical skin-care line but also very elegant, feminine, and sensual.

Skin is the largest organ of the body (sorry, guys). It's made of two layers, epidermis and dermis. Starting as young as our twenties, skin begins to become less firm and elastic as collagen and elastin production slow down in the dermis. Also, less oil may be produced in the skin, leading to dryness.

Skin ages through two processes: genetically programmed aging and environmental aging. Genetically programmed aging is inherited; it's what our cells are biologically programmed to do. Along with natural aging, we all experience some degree of environmental aging. That's the extra damage the skin endures from its surroundings, mostly from the sun. (Smoking is also a killer, not just to your lungs but also to your skin.) This damage collects under the skin long before it becomes visible on the surface. The environmental damage will hurry the effects of genetically programmed aging and make them much more severe. Part of the reason is that aging epidermis no longer sloughs off easily. In addition, environmental aging can be responsible for the majority of skin changes that make us look older—brown spots, surface roughness, fine wrinkles, blotchiness, and increased skin sensitivity.

Your skin wants to rejuvenate every twenty-one days. But as you age, it doesn't do this as well as it did when you were young. It needs a bit of help. One of the secrets to youthful-looking skin is retinol. Retinol is vitamin A and it accelerates the rejuvenating process by speeding up the sloughing off of the top layer of the epidermis. As it does, it eases the appearance of blotchiness, age spots, uneven skin tone, and redness. You're literally coming up with new baby butt skin.

One of the big things that folks don't realize is that when retinol is exposed to light and air it's like leaving a carton of milk out on the counter at night—it can spoil. So all those expensive products that you may have in your bathroom that contain retinol are becoming less effective every time they're exposed to light and air.

It's also important for aging skin to be retexturized on a weekly basis. This is important because your pores are like baggies. As you get older, skin loses its collagen, its elasticity. Your pores can fill up with old makeup and dead skin and get bigger and bigger. So you've got to clean them out.

Of course, a major skin-care tip is to stay out of the sun as much as possible. Since I have very light skin I have always tried to avoid the sun, even before we knew it was bad for us. We should all use a sunscreen with at least SPF 15 every day on all parts of the skin that may be exposed to the sun. Even with sunscreen, try to avoid the midday sun (between 10 A.M. and 4 P.M.). The sun's rays are very direct at this time of day and much more damaging. Believe me, skin cancer can be deadly. Tanning beds are not a safe alternative. I've heard of women actually getting addicted to tanning beds. They get a serotonin glow with the tan. My dermatologist tells me he treats women with skin cancer who are still using the tanning bed. Take a tip from the stars—use tan in a can like Sally Hansen if you want a brown glow. The leg spray in the summer is better than wearing panty hose. Jergens Natural Glow Daily Moisturizer will add a slightly golden shade too.

What's good for your body and brain is also good for your skin. So all you can do for your physical health, as described in Chapter 8, will also show on your face. And don't forget to drink plenty of water. Skin needs lots of hydration to glow. (Your eyes do too, by the way. They can really dry out as you age. I find that the viscous Refresh eyedrops are the best.)

## Naps, Nips, and Tucks

"Money can't buy you happiness, but it can pay for the plastic surgery."

—JOAN RIVERS

As we get older, lack of sleep really shows on the face, so don't neglect the importance of a good night's sleep. Most of us need seven to nine hours every night for our bodies and minds to repair and recharge.

If you don't get enough sleep, your body produces less of the hormones that regulate your appetite, causing you to crave sweets and salty carbs. Studies show that overweight individuals are often suffering from a lack of sleep. And lack of sleep can even bring on depression.

If you have trouble sleeping, avoid caffeine (watch out for chocolate—it's in there, too) and alcohol. Both interfere with sleep. Don't exercise within three hours of going to bed. It revs you up. Try to go to bed at the same time each night to train your mind and body to a regular schedule. Do a relaxing ritual beforehand—take a warm bath, listen to relaxing music. Lower the lights in your bedroom three hours before you retire. Try repeating a little meditation to yourself before going to sleep, such as, "I will wake up tomorrow feeling refreshed and energetic." If you can't fall asleep within fifteen minutes, try reading or some other relaxing activity. Being well rested can make all the difference in looking great and having an enjoyable, productive day.

No chapter on looking good as we get older should avoid the topic of plastic surgery. Of course, dear reader, I know you are wondering if I've had a face-lift. The answer is yes. I did it years ago because I was thirty-eight when I entered the "looks are everything" world of show business.

I don't think plastic surgery is wrong. Craniofacial plastic surgery, for cleft palates or accident victims, for instance, is life changing. It's marvelous stuff. My criteria is: What is your reason? Will it look natural? I'm still glad I had it done. In today's world, as much as we wish it weren't true, appearance counts.

However, I must tell you that a face-lift is a more serious procedure than I expected.

I am concerned about today's overuse of plastic surgery and about trying to live up to impossible images of perfection depicted on TV and in magazines. Did you know it's possible to become a plastic surgery addict? I once heard a man on *Oprah* talk about working three jobs to pay for his wife's constant plastic surgeries. That's not okay. There's also the story of a school superintendent in Atlanta, Georgia, who embezzled money from the school system to pay for a face-lift. She is now behind bars serving time. This is very sad to me. Recently, a young college student, Kacey Long, was a guest on my Hallmark show, *Naomi's New Morning*. She came on the show to talk about her experience with breast implants and to warn others about the possible dangers with side effects. Kacey longed to have the full-figured look she had seen so often in magazines, so she saved her money and was able eventually to get the implants. Soon afterward she fell ill and was diagnosed with fibromyalgia and rheumatoid arthritis, which her doctors suspect are a result of the implants. She has since had the implants removed but still suffers from the side effects.

When you have a healthy self-concept, some plastic surgery is not a problem. But a scalpel is not a magic wand. When people use it to contrive a false self-image or to look like someone else, it can lead to depression and other negative consequences. If you think it's going to solve problems in your life, then you are delusional. If your looks, for instance, are the most important thing to your mate, that relationship is ill-fated.

People in Hollywood often overdo it. Think of all those celebrities who look like they're under constant g forces. If you do plan to have plastic surgery, be sure to get referrals from people you trust. Find someone who is board certified (you can call the American Board of Plastic Surgery at 215-587-9322 or check online at www.abplsurg.org). Ask about how many times a month they perform the procedure you're considering and how many surgeries a day they do. If they say more than three, chances are someone else is doing the prep or finishing work. You want someone who will be with you the whole time. Make sure you ask about risks and find out if they will do redos for free if you need a touch-up. Pay attention to all the pre-op literature. And then make sure you know what you have to do postsurgery to avoid complications and get the best results. Think through how you'll delegate tasks while you're recuperating.

Be whoever you are, acknowledge your individuality, and make the best of your qualities. As Anne Lamott says, "You celebrate what works and you take tender care of what doesn't, with lotion, polish, and kindness."

## Saving Face

"Ya gots to work with what you gots to work with."
—STEVIE WONDER

The older I get, the less makeup and the more underwear I wear. I wore too much makeup all my life. People tried to tell me all the time I didn't need to wear all that makeup. My own daughters most of all: "Mom, you're wearing too much makeup."

When Larry and I first started living together, I even wore makeup to bed! I look back at that time now and I just can't understand my lack of self-confidence. What an amazing amount of time and negative energy I expended. Finally, I got that I didn't need to cover myself up, but to enhance what was already there.

Now I mainly just wear makeup when I'm working. I call it the plain truth.

There are a few tricks in learning how to use makeup well, especially as our skin ages. Have you noticed that powder makes lines and wrinkles more noticeable? Try this: First use a rich moisturizer before applying liquid foundation. Then blot with a Kleenex instead of using powder. This removes excess foundation so you don't have a waxy or shiny look. If you have oily skin, pick oil-free makeup.

For lines around your eyes, make sure your concealer is not too thick, since it can actually make wrinkles look worse. Also, make sure your foundation matches your skin color exactly. Blend foundation to the hairline and chin line and make sure there's no noticeable line. Does it disappear after it's applied? Become greasy? Change color? If so, change products. Also, remember not to use it on your neck or it will end up on your clothes. (If you do get it on your clothes, rubbing alcohol will remove it.)

Since your skin gets drier as you age, go for the cream rouge. (When I was growing up, color was called rouge, the French word for "red." Then it became powder blush or cheek color.)

As for eyebrows, you want a brow that is slightly thicker toward the nose, arches over the center, and thins out. Never use liquid eye-liner. Too starkly obvious. I use a soft pencil and then take a Q-tip to smudge it a little to avoid a strong line.

And remember: Pul-leeeze no blue eye shadow or other outrageous colors. Too much color and you'll look like a clown. Try the neutral tones. They're supposed to notice you, not the makeup. Watch out for iridescent eye shadows, which include ground-up seashells, since many women are allergic to seashells. Eyelid skin is very, very thin and so this type of shadow often makes your eyes swell and run. (Plus it accentuates wrinkles.)

When it comes to lipstick color, the thinner your lips, the more intense the color can be. If you use lip liner, be sure the liner isn't darker than your lipstick and blend the line. Apply lip glosses and greasy lipsticks only in the center of your lips—they can easily bleed into the lines around your mouth. Restylane has replaced collagen as a filler and is often used to fill in those vertical lines around the upper lips. It's expensive but available through injections by a cosmetic surgeon.

Putting on makeup is mostly trial and error. You want to come up with what makes you feel and look good, which may mean modifying your regimen as you age. Always, the aim is to look natural and smooth rather than artificial or painted on. That's where the importance of blending comes in. Use a makeup sponge or warm fingertip to blend.

Be sure to consider how your hair color complements your skin tone. And how about that hairstyle? Does it need an update? Are you stuck in the past with a poofy 'do or a perm that was last in style in the eighties? Look around and pay attention to what's current. Find a style that flatters you in this decade.

Trying to look or act younger than you are "is silly, very silly." The more realistic you are, the happier you'll be, says the Dalai Lama.

# Clothes Make the Woman

When it comes to clothes, I like what May Sarton said about the older I get, the more I become who I really am. After she turned fifty, Oprah gave away a thousand outfits (actually, she auctioned them off for charity) because they did not make her feel "alive." That's what dressing well as we age is all about—feeling alive in whatever you're wearing. Finally we can stop paying attention to styles and trends and enjoy clothes that suit us personally. I don't do bows, ruffles, or polka dots. Not gonna do it, even if they are the hottest things in fashion.

Dressing well is about finding clothes that are the right color and style for your body type and coloring. Have you had enough of dressing like everyone else? I was at Saks Fifth Avenue in New York watching women ogling $1,500 purses. They were going to spend an absurd amount of money on a trendy designer bag because they believed somehow it would get them into an exclusive club. Why else would you pay $1,500 for a purse? It's just a purse! The retailers get you twice. They get your money and they take your individuality. À la Stepford Wives.

When you are really happy with who you are, you buy only what you need or what you absolutely love. For instance, I travel so much that I have to carry a briefcase and a purse. I wouldn't make it with heavy designer bags. I want something that's light, has a lot of compartments, and has a zipper for safety.

If you have children or grandchildren, ask them how you look. I benefit from Wy and Ashley's wardrobe tips. Once while Ashley was picking out some gowns for the Oscars with Samantha McMillen, her wardrobe gal, I took advantage of the opportunity and said, "Okay, girls, hit me with it. Tell me what I'm doing wrong fashionwise." In unison they yelled, "You match too much."

Guilty as charged by the fashion police! Probably some genetic predisposition, because my mother does it too. I'm keenly aware of that every time I'm around her now. I'll offer, "You know, instead of being red from head to toe, can you throw in another color?" Have you noticed that matching is a problem with many women over fifty? We always believed in matching handbag, shoes, and jewelry.

Reasons for my matching compulsion include that it's easier to pack stuff that all goes together. But it's also because I haven't been pausing to check out the whole look in a full-length mirror. Go get a full-length mirror, girls. Spend the last five minutes before you walk out of the door seeing yourself in the mirror like everyone else will see you. It will be obvious that the necklace is overpowering, that those earrings with that necklace are too much, etc. You have to look at the whole picture.

(Know how you know if you've reached middle age? Joey Green and Alan Corcoran have written a funny little book about the clues: You and your spouse wear color-coordinated outfits; you look better in long sleeves; you'd rather buy control-top panty hose than go to the gym; you've switched from baby oil and iodine to SPF 45 sunscreen; you need a Weed-wacker to trim the hair growing from your nose, ears, and eyebrows; you've realized that all those geeky people in Bermuda shorts walking around Disney World include you.)

When going out in public, consider the occasion and ask yourself what texture or color or slight detail gives you personality and individual taste but doesn't look like you're trying too hard. When it comes to choosing clothes it's all about (1) finding the right shapes, styles, and colors and (2) downplaying your flaws and accentuating your best. If you're small-framed like me, stay away from heavily textured fabrics with large buttons. They will overpower you. However, if you're big boned, you might do better with the heavy fabrics and strong details, 'cause delicate fabrics and tiny buttons could make you look silly. If you have a thick

## NAOMI'S NO-NOS

As we age, if you can't be a good example, you may be a horrible warning. I've learned to stay far away from

- rings on every finger (attention, nurses, this goes for you too)

- panty hose with sandals (I would use the tan in a can if I needed it for coloring)

- humongous eyeglasses

- big fancy earrings with jogging suits

- colors like pastel blue and pink that make me look like I've reverted to childhood

- holiday-themed sweaters and sweatshirts—Christmas, Easter, or Halloween decorations

- hats at night

- no "outfits" (choose pieces that go well together but aren't matching). Mix, don't match. Matching is old-fashioned.

- tight clothes that show every bulge and totally shapeless clothes that look like tents

- T-shirts, halter tops

waist, wear your blouse out. Hippy? Wear longer jackets. Got fabulous legs? Wear shorter skirts to show them off. I've never found kneecaps attractive, so all my skirts are either at the middle of or almost to the bottom of the knee.

Consider your wardrobe requirements as you decide your makeover. For example, I'm full breasted, and after seeing enough photos, it finally dawned on me I don't look good in T-shirts or sweaters. Blouses are better. Structure is a must. I like collars that give you a V above cleavage. With my facial structure, I look much better with a definitive shoulder line. Since I don't have broad shoulders, I sometimes sew Velcro strips in my blouses so I can attach shoulder pads to create a bit more of a horizontal line. I believe I look best in three-quarter sleeves and a top that goes in at the waist and flares out over my hips. I like to wear what we used to call flood pants, crop pants. But if I was very much shorter I wouldn't wear them because they chop short women off. It's all because of a full-length mirror that I was able to figure this stuff out. Look at yourself in the mirror and study it a bit. Consider that something you looked good in when you were young may not suit you now.

As Gypsy Rose Lee admitted, "I have everything I had twenty years ago, only it's all a little lower." Go to a good department store and get fitted with the right bra. You might also want to consider those body shapers that help give hips and thighs a smoother line. And don't forget good posture—the straighter you stand, the better you look and the less your bosom will be at your navel!

If you haven't already, you should seriously consider getting your colors done. Color analysis is a way to find the colors that complement your skin, eye, and hair color. You end up with a swatch of a wide variety of hues that flatter your coloring and harmonize with each other. If you use your colors to buy clothes, it's much easier to wind up with a wardrobe in which things go together.

Color analysis is based on the seasons:

- Winters have blue or pink undertones to their complexion. Skin is pale white, yellowish-olive, or dark. Hair is usually brown or black and eyes are usually dark. Many Asians and African Americans fall into this category.

- Summers also have blue or pink skin undertones, but their skin is pale and pink. Summers are usually blondes or brunettes with pale eyes.

- Autumns have golden undertones. They are often redheads and brunettes with golden brown eyes.

- Spring complexions have golden undertones and are usually creamy white or peach. Spring people generally have light blonde or strawberry red hair, freckles, rosy cheeks, and blue or green eyes.

You can get your colors done by a color analyst or through the internet for free at www.homemakingcottage.com/woman/dressing_up .htm.

## Stepping Out on the Right Foot

"You'd have to shoot me before I'd put on stilettos."
—MOLLY IVINS

As we get older, footwear becomes a new frontier. We don't want to wear ankle breakers, yet shoes for "older" women sometimes look orthopedically corrective. A girlfriend had on such a pair. So I said teasingly, "How long do you have to wear those?" Friends don't let friends wear ugly shoes.

TV's Jane Pauley and I were discussing ridiculously high and uncomfortable shoes. "Why the heck are sensible women teetering around on these implausibly uncomfortable stilettos?" I asked. Jane's retort was "Because you can't find attractive shoes."

Check out the Dr. Taryn Rose brand. She was an orthopedic surgeon who's developed an attractive line. You can find them at Nordstrom and Neiman Marcus, as well as online at www.shoescentral.net or www.zappos.com.

The size and contour of your feet change as you grow older. It's best to measure them at the end of the day because when you have been upright all day, your feet are the largest. And don't forget, one foot is larger than the other, so make sure the larger foot feels good in the shoe.

Just like when you were a teen and you started to individuate and experiment to find your style, as you mature you need to do the same. Once as I was visiting Dolly Parton, I asked, "Now that you've turned sixty are you going to alter your image?" "Oh, yeah," she chirped. "It's going to get worse!"

## Your Turn Now

- Have you been neglecting your looks? What could you do right now to make yourself feel better inside and out?

- Do you think vanity is a sin? How many times a day do you look in the mirror?

- Whom do you know who tries too hard to look young? Do you feel pressured to dress a certain way or look a certain way— makeup or no makeup, for instance—from anyone in your family?

- What's your favorite outfit and why?

- Take a good look in a full-length mirror. Have you updated your style in the past ten years? What two things would you like to change about your looks?

- Would you consider shopping in new stores?

- Can you accept a compliment? Next time someone says you look good, rather than brushing it off, say, "Thank you." Really receive it!

I want to go on living even after my death.
And therefore I am grateful to God
For giving this gift . . .
Of expressing all that is in me.
—ANNE FRANK

## 10 | *It's a Wonderful Life:* Grieving, God, and Passing on Values (as Well as Valuables)

EVERY CHAPTER BEGINS with a personal story of how I learned from a crisis or mistake. I'll close with a bang—this is one I've never told anyone.

On Christmas Day 2005, in Ashley and Dario's house at the family table, I almost died in front of the people I love most.

The day began so joyfully! We met at Wy and Roach's, where we enjoyed Santa's gifts to Elijah and Grace, then moved over to Ashley and Dario's home. Ashley had festively decorated and set a lovely table for our delicious dinner. I plunked down my usual vitamins on my place at the table. Being very knowledgeable about supplements and herbs, Ashley gave me a nickel-sized vitamin C and zinc lozenge for my sore throat. Laughing and talking, completely at ease in that wonderfully warm and fuzzy family scene, I didn't bother to look down as I grabbed what I expected to be a vitamin. The minute I took a swig of water to wash it down, a large lozenge sealed my windpipe completely. With my trachea blocked, the water spurted back out my nose and mouth. I bolted upright in terror. Seated directly across from me, Wy locked eyes with me and hollered, "Mom's not okay." My arms were flailing as I frantically pointed to my throat. Everyone's chairs pushed back in unison as they rushed around me.

If you've ever had your airway cut off, you know it's one of the most terrifying events a human being can experience. Wy yelled, "Do you need to be Heimliched?" I nodded and Larry performed the maneuver twice. Ashley rushed to get me warm water as she calculated it might hasten the softening and melting of the large throat lozenge. (It's made to dissolve slowly in the mouth.) Meanwhile, Wy was extending her palms forward, frozen in horror, praying loudly for me to breathe again.

It was a most unimaginable situation. Larry, Ashley, Dario, Wy, Roach, Elijah, and Grace stood helpless in front of me. "I can't die on Christmas Day at Ashley's dinner table in front of my family," I pleaded with God. The Heimlich failed to eject the lozenge, but I felt it turn a tad on its side. Ash calmly insisted I sip the warm water. Although it was counterintuitive, I took tiny sips. Some water sputtered back up. She urged me to keep sipping. I'd been without air for at least one and a half minutes. Feeling light-headed, I was starting to lose consciousness when suddenly I got the slightest whisper of air! This gave me motivation to keep sipping the warm water. The dissolving lozenge began ever so slowly to slip down my throat.

As soon as we were certain I could breathe again, Larry burst into tears. Everyone joined in a circle as Ashley led us in a gratitude blessing. Powerful stuff. I lost track of how long we all just sat together hugging and calming down. We then consoled wide-eyed Elijah and Grace as our conversation turned to reviewing how everyone performed and how important it is to remain calm in any life-threatening scenario. The doctor later found I had a broken rib from Larry's Heimlich maneuver, but at least I didn't choke to death in front of my family on Christmas.

As we retired to the living room resplendent with tree and presents, we reflected that this would be a Christmas to be remembered! Not for what we got, but for what we already had.

This dramatic family scare provides the concept for this last chapter. As you ponder making out a will, deciding to whom you'll leave your material valuables, you should consider something more important: How will you bequeath your values?

Materialism's never been my thing. Sure, Wy, Ash, and my grandkids will inherit all my material possessions, but aging gratefully has taught me to be more concerned with letting my loved ones know how much I love them. I want to pass down, in an ethical will, my values.

What are your most valuable material treasures? If your house was on fire, what would you grab? One of my first objects would be a cheap pink polyester pincushion proclaiming, "I love you, Mom." Wy and I were embroiled in a hellacious argument on our tour bus one night. About 3 A.M. at a truck stop in Texas she bought the tiny pincushion and slipped it under the door to my room. Of course, that was the end of our fight. It now sits next to an equally valuable brown clay vase Ashley created when she was eight. My daddy's Bible is very precious to me also.

As I'm writing this chapter, middle Tennessee experienced devastating tornadoes, killing twelve people. Other home owners and business owners shown on the local TV news lost everything. Standing amid the desolation and rubble, they declared they're grateful no one in their family was harmed. They value the people in their lives more than their possessions.

## *When You Reach the Top, Send the Elevator Back Down to Get Others*

"I know God will not give me anything I can't handle. I just wish that He didn't trust me so much."

—MOTHER TERESA

Holocaust victim Anne Frank had no valuables, but what she wrote about in her diary to this day makes us think twice about our own values and mortality.

You may have decided who will get your valuables—your money, your property, even your organs. But what about your values? Values as well as valuables are meant to be passed on to the next generation. One of the best legacies baby boomers can leave to the next generation is to teach them to value and respect their elders.

Erik Erikson called this stage of life "generativity," the caring for the generations that will come after us by connecting to those younger and passing on the value of our wisdom. Here's how Harvard researcher George E. Vaillant put it in his book *Aging Well:* "The old are put on earth to nurture the young." Mentoring is the gift from your lifetime. The best gift, because it keeps on giving. Check out the website for Elder Wisdom Circle, which offers wisdom from 250 cybergrandparents whom youngsters can email with their questions.

This concept greatly benefits baby boomers as well. It turns out that recognizing and meeting the need for generativity is one of the crucial factors in happy, healthy, grateful aging. For the past fifty years, doctors at the Harvard Medical School have been studying 824 people to discover the secrets of mental and physical health. You've read in the preceding chapters much of what researchers have discovered from them about successful aging. But the last remaining one is this: People who aged well emotionally, physically, and mentally found ways after fifty to guide the younger generations as mentors, coaches, and consultants.

There are movies about these acts of meaning and purpose. Think of *The Karate Kid, Searching for Bobby Fischer, Finding Forrester, In Good Company.* (Hey, when are we going to see ones starring women?)

When you provide emotional empowerment or some gift of your experience to another, it's spiritual alchemy. It's a transfer of positive energy from you to another who may not even be aware he or she needs it at the time. Generativity is unselfish. From this special place, we offer the value of our experiences so that others will benefit from what we've already lived. We're no longer looking for a payback or an award. We're not here to show them how to follow in our footsteps but to offer up ideas so they can become more fully themselves. We're cool if young folks take or leave our advice. The point is to offer. Ironically, those who are the most generative describe that in giving they also receive. They've seen enough and are therefore wise enough to remain open to learning something from those they're helping. Generativity becomes a two-way street.

The point of the movie *Pay It Forward* is that when someone does something nice for you, you don't pay the favor back; you pay it forward by helping someone else. That's the essence of generativity. You have been helped in ways seen and unseen since the day you were born. Now it's your turn to pay it forward.

The hugely best-selling book *Tuesdays with Morrie* is the true story of a dying college professor who decided to make generativity his final project. Tuesday meetings with former student Mitch Albom became the center point of his last days as the value of his life wisdom became a human textbook. Student Mitch learned how to live more fully by learning how one dies with dignity. He then tweaked the lens through which he viewed his own life so it became more clearly in focus from then on.

As we age, we pay less and less attention to parenting and career. We find ourselves freer to become concerned about larger issues—freedom, justice, our community, the environment, health, and wellness for all people. The specific issue that captures our individual attention has everything to do with our personal history. The events we've personally struggled with and learned from give us practical wisdom we should pass on.

I met a woman who exemplifies this type of generativity: the Honorable Shirin Ebadi, the 2003 Nobel Peace Prize winner. Sixty-year-old Iranian Shirin Ebadi is a devout Muslim. A lawyer and former judge until women were barred from being judges, she has advocated for an interpretation of Islamic law consistent with democracy and equality for women and religious minorities. The Iranian government has jailed her many times, but that has never stopped her. In one of her most famous cases, Shirin represented a woman whose child had been taken from her and died in foster care. Despite enormous pressure, Judge Ebadi led a campaign against violence against children and managed for the first time to convince legislators to criminalize such violence. She now lectures on human rights at Tehran University and around the world.

Coming up with ways to pass on wisdom helps make sense of our past hardships. I'm available to share what I know from my bout with hepatitis C with those who have been diagnosed with it. This connection gives meaning, enjoyment, and satisfaction to this important phase of aging. It "crowns our lives with worth and nobility," as Rabbi Zalman Schachter-Shalomi says.

According to a survey of youth by the Horatio Alger Foundation, after drugs and peer pressure, a decline in values is the third worst influence on kids. When asked to name a hero, the most common answer was, "I don't have one." Get your attention? Do you have a grandchild, a niece, a nephew, or a neighbor who's a child of a single mother? In 2006, 50 percent of all American kids will at some point live in a single-parent home. Some of the ways you can pass on your wisdom could be volunteering in a classroom, at Big Brothers and Sisters, teaching reading at the local library, or coaching on a basketball court. It could be by audio- or videotaping your life lessons for your grandchildren or nieces and nephews. Know how to play an instrument? Teach someone who otherwise would never learn.

Ashley had just flown back from Africa, where she'd been volunteering for two weeks in her role as global ambassador for Youth AIDS. The stress of witnessing human misery and the extreme rigors of travel had made her feel yucky.

Although just getting home, she asked Larry to drive her to the city council meeting in Franklin. Weak and out of it, she was still determined to protest a proposed housing development on the site of a Civil War battlefield. Ashley values preserving our historic community. They stopped at Wy's to pick up eight-year-old Gracie, who had crafted a sign proclaiming, "Franklin is special." I stood in the driveway watching these three generations head off to the meeting and smiled in recognition that the torch had been passed on to Gracie. And oh, yes, the proposal to develop on the historic site was defeated!

My legacy consists of six essential beliefs:

1   I believe I can connect with and honor God by using my talents to manifest just about anything my hearts desires. I truly believe that all things are possible when we believe, behave, and ask. So go ahead and take God up on His promises. Acknowledge that your birthright is to become a winner.

2   No matter your age, in order to achieve whatever goal or thing you're wanting, come up with a time line and put together a practical plan infused with wild imagination.

3   Constantly choose higher awareness by understanding that every issue is actually a spiritual problem with a spiritual solution. Ask: What is this prickly situation trying to teach me?

4   Realize that when you can't control your circumstances, you still get to choose your reaction. Take comfort in knowing that this is your point of personal power. It transforms every circumstance into something manageable.

5   Breathe deeply and relax into the moment. Slow down, simplify, and be kind.

6   Your life right now is a result of all the choices you've made so far. When you are willing to change your mind, your entire world will improve.

These six messages infuse all my books and speaking engagements, and my Hallmark Channel show, *Naomi's New Morning*. My values are revealed naturally in day-to-day interactions with friends, family, and strangers. What you are reading right now is my ethical will made public.

Now what are the essential messages you want to leave behind as your legacy? Where and how are you going to share them? With family? Younger colleagues? The latchkey kid down the street lacking a role model? Write them down and include them in your will.

The Bible says, "As you sow, so shall ye reap." Some call it karma. Our actions really do come back full circle. For years, people have related how they played the Judds' song "Grandpa" at their grandfather's funeral. Recently my own family was sitting in a church in Garner, North Carolina, at Larry's father's funeral. All around us were Ralph's adult children, grandchildren, and great-grandchildren. As they carried the casket out, they played "Grandpa."

Our true "social security" is found in being social with others. As we age, we should socialize with younger generations. Nurture and bond with them, for it is they who will make the next choices for the good of all—or not. When we choose to keep on giving from our experiences, we have influence on the future.

## The Final Frontier

"Death is not extinguishing the light; it is putting out the lamp because dawn has come."

—RABINDRANATH TAGORE

Death is our society's last taboo. We talk about all kinds of things in public that we shouldn't, except death. Not only will talking about death not kill you, it may even help you live more fully. But since most of us can't begin to face the reality of our own death, we avoid it like the plague. Have you done any planning for it? Do you avoid conversation about it?

It's time for us baby boomers to come out of the closet! And with eighty-five million Americans over fifty, it's a mighty large closet. We owe it to ourselves and our loved ones to do this right. The great psychologist Erik Erikson, the pioneer of adult development, stated that one of the key jobs of the old is to show the young how not to fear death. You and I can do that by choosing to bring this most fascinating of all topics out into the open. As with any emotional issue, the journey must begin within us. We can start by identifying and working through whatever fear is in ourselves.

Much of our fear of death is due simply to lack of exposure. Nowadays, instead of dying in their own home, people get whisked away to other places—first the hospital or nursing home, and then the funeral home. And we avoid those who are dying because we're uncomfortable. We don't know how to handle the unpleasant situation, and we don't want to face our own impending death. But the more we can learn about the process of dying, the better we can choose how we want to go through it.

That's exactly what happened to Wynonna. She benefited by experiencing the gentle passing of TV producer Gene Weed, Dick Clark's partner. Gene organized the Academy of Country Music Awards show. When he was dying, Gene asked to see us.

Wy, who used to have trouble even being around sick people, was extremely anxious. I remembered how on a trip to Columbus in 1984 for a concert, I took her to the Rainbow Children's Hospital so we could cheer up the kids in pediatrics. She went in the bathroom and threw up. Now fast-forward to seeing Gene on his deathbed. Fortunately, by then she had really matured and handled it as well as I did.

Choosing not to die in a hospital, Gene was under hospice care at his home in the San Fernando Valley. We found him lying in a hospital bed in the middle of the living room, hooked up to a morphine drip. It was ominous. I lowered the bed rail and told him I was so glad our lives had intersected. Even though he was in some pain, he groggily smiled. I reminisced about the milestones of our time together, when Wy and I cohosted the show and won the ACMs Duo award eight years in a row. Then he motioned for Larry and whispered, "You take care of her and I'll see you both on the other side." Wy and I were in the process of recording a duet for her millennium CD at the time called "That's What Makes You Strong." We sang it for him and later dedicated it to Gene on the CD. He passed over to the other side just a few days later.

This was a pivotal experience for Wynonna. Not only did she come face-to-face with her own fear of death, but Roach, not yet her husband, showed his faith and goodness as he comforted her through it. She says this is when she fell in love with him.

As Wy and I discussed this event, she came to the conclusion that when you choose to confront your fear of death, you feel free and empowered. Whenever you're afraid, the first step is to name the fear. It will diminish its hold on you when you call it by name, step back, and observe it objectively.

I've had the sacred privilege of being with other human beings as they were making the passage. As an RN, I've been witness when someone takes their last breath—expire—just as I've seen babies take their first breath—inspire.

I don't know how I could have survived all that's happened to me without a strong spiritual foundation. My connection to God has helped me survive abuse, a near-fatal illness, family challenges, and the death of loved ones. It's not about how we look, what we have, or any of the success trappings by which society tries to rate us. Therefore, I don't fear growing older. I trust that everything after death is already taken care of. When I say God holds my whole world together, I mean it.

How about you? As you get older, your friends and family are too.

Losing loved ones is inevitable. I describe it as feeling like you're in an earthquake. There's a loss of control and you feel as though all you ever knew and trusted is destroyed along with the persistent fear and knowledge it will happen again. The aftershocks of sadness and doubt are tiny deaths in themselves, rooted in thoughts of the past and future. Only the present moment actually holds peace. Your senses are there to tune you into mindfulness of the present. Some of the ways to help you stay more focused in the present are massage, movies and books, having friends close by, being in nature, expressing yourself through writing or music, or simply vicariously enjoying others' joys or passions. Unfortunately, I know what it's like to feel humbled and totally diminished by loss and betrayal. I felt like a tiny sparrow shivering on a high lonesome branch looking down in complete silence and wondering how the world was still turning. But I learned that even though our emotions may be like a frigid frozen lake, there are warmer currents flowing underneath.

A spiritual framework can bring great solace by helping you face the inevitability of death. Facing death square on also helps us strip down to see clearly what our priorities and values are. It gets us thinking about what life lessons and memories we want to leave so that our own existence will continue to matter after we are gone. Our earthly experience in this physical body can be over any minute. Let's externalize this awareness by planning how to leave a legacy while we still have the time.

**"We believe life is measured in memories, not years."**
—MAKE A WISH FOUNDATION

# Soul Survivor

"A grandfather was walking through his yard when he heard his granddaughter repeating the alphabet in a tone of voice that sounded like a prayer. He asked her what she was doing. The little girl explained: 'I'm praying, but I can't think of exactly the right words, so I'm just saying all the letters, and God will put them together for me, because He knows what I'm thinking.' "
—CHARLES B. VAUGHAN

Among the many important cultural changes attributed to baby boomers is the way their spiritual practices diverged from the way their World War II parents worshipped. As spiritual seekers, some boomers dropped out of traditional congregations, demanding more, creating new forms of worship. Responsible for culture wars on social issues, they expect relevance in ideological issues. Whether it's checking out Eastern religions, or returning to their classic practices, baby boomers have realized that money, power, and sex couldn't fulfill them. They even invented megachurches to downplay topics of sin and hell, instead celebrating positive psychology and joyful music. Fragmentation, pragmatism, and hopefulness are baby boomers' spiritual contributions.

"Well, I certainly don't believe God's a woman, because if He were, men would be the ones walking around wearing high heels, taking Midol, and having their upper lips waxed."
—DIXIE CARTER IN *DESIGNING WOMEN*

When I was young, I listened intently to Sunday school teachers explain the miracles in the Bible. I enjoyed trusting in the intriguing mystery that God is way beyond human understanding. Broader and deeper than anyone's intellect. As an adult, my interest continued to expand into the spirit/mind/body connection. I've sought out renowned physicists, chemists, and psychiatrists who see God through science. They explained that the universe is so exquisitely elegant that there has to be a prime intelligent source behind it. I highly recommend my friend Dr. Francis Collins's brilliant new book *The Language of God: A Scientist Presents Evidence for Belief.* (As head of the NIH Human Genome Project, Dr. Collins decoded the genome and explores bioethics.)

I don't need a scientist to convince me that there is a God. I've always known that there was something more than myself, my family, my neighborhood, and my hometown of Ashland, Kentucky. We willingly went to Sunday school and church every week. I liked dressing up and going together as a family on a special day.

It was the stories that really drew me in, the parables and the teachings of Jesus Christ. One Saturday at the Twenty-first Street market, Mom ran into my Sunday school teacher, who chuckled, "Well, I've got to hurry home and prepare for Naomi's inevitable questions in Sunday school."

My faith was tested when I was diagnosed with terminal hepatitis C. I didn't go through the "why me?" phase. Partly because during that time a spiritual mentor appeared. When the student is ready, the teacher will appear. He taught me that we're all spiritual beings having a human experience. That thought kicked me forward into a broader realm of awareness. I blurted, "What? Stop the world! Say that again." Then I relaxed into the realization that if all I have is God, that's still enough. Whenever I feel helpless, I'm still not hopeless. I may be overwhelmed, but I'm not overcome.

Don't you long to feel whole? Wholeness is an abstract thought.

It's a symbol of qualities like self-awareness, compassion, and connection to God for a higher emotional state.

Do you know you can find spiritual comfort in trying times? Belief in God encourages us to try harder and comforts us when we deal with pain, illness, infirmity, and impending death. It keeps us from sinking down into despair and assures us we're not alone. Faith steers us toward better daily lifestyle choices, gives us social support through church activities, and reduces stress. It provides shape to the simplest activities we enjoy throughout our days and adds meaning to our lives overall.

Research has shown that people with strong religious connections live, on average, seven years longer than those who don't, and have greater mental, emotional, and physical health. They are less depressed, anxious, and suicidal, and better able to cope with divorce, illness, and death of a loved one. One study found that church attendance was more related to satisfaction with health than age, race, education, gender, marital status, or recent hospitalization. Another one shows that people who believe in God experience less pain from advanced cancer than nonbelievers.

In the past ten years or so, there has been much research done on the effects of prayer. Mind-body guru Herbert Benson of Harvard Medical School has found that prayer lowers blood pressure and reduces pain in cancer patients. Prayer has also been found to reduce stress and speed recovery from illness. In one study, terminally ill people who were prayed for visited the doctor less frequently, were hospitalized less often, and had much improvement in mood over those who were not. Some studies have found such effects even when the patients don't know they are being prayed for! Dr. Dale Matthews, author of *Faith Factor* and an expert on prayer, taught me that patients do better when their doctors pray with them. Dr. Dale encourages us to choose doctors who are believers and are willing to pray with us.

As a Christian, I believe in God the Father and in Jesus Christ, His Son. I realize of course that not everyone does. Ninety-five percent of Americans acknowledge a power greater than themselves. I believe there are many paths but only one journey. The most significant difference between Christianity and other religions, the event that sets us apart from others, is the Resurrection. We believe in a risen Savior. When I'm having trouble waking up and getting out of bed, I think how hard it must have been to rise from the dead and get out of a rocked-over, sealed tomb.

It's critical here to take note of the difference between religion and spirituality. Religion is about beliefs, doctrine, sacred texts, and tradition. Unfortunately, historically speaking, religion's strict dogma tends to divide us. Spirituality is about deep feelings and enlightening experiences that are unique to each individual. For most, spirituality is discovered through religion. But if this hasn't been true for you yet, I encourage you to find ways to explore and connect to your spirituality. Growing old without deep faith can leave one despondent and fatalistic.

When I pray, it's like what Robert De Niro taught Ashley about acting: "The words in the script [prayer] are just the boat to get you into the water [connect to God]." Prayer is an inner opening to God. When I pray, I become aware I'm in a contract with God and taking Him up on His promise. Here's an example of a prayer I use at times:

> Father, by whom all things are made and without whom
> nothing ever was, is right now, or ever can be, I come boldly into
> the throne room to beseech You and to enter into an intimate
> conversation with You because of what my personal savior Jesus
> did on the cross at Calvary, His blood that was shed and so sealed
> a contract, a legal binding contract so that I may inherit and

fulfill my birthright. Therefore I now open my heart, mind, and spirit to come boldly before You in my time of need.

Then I pray for whatever I need. I confidently ask for help to become my highest self and for the highest good. I've turned my need over to God. You may consider prayer as your portal to enlightenment, the contact point between your human thoughts and the Ultimate Divine Mind. Prayer creates molds to shape what you're yearning for. A well-posed question has half the answer in it.

To me, praying is like taking your broken wristwatch to a repair shop. You have to hand it over to the expert to be fixed. That doesn't mean I don't have a sense of responsibility to act on what I need to be doing. It's an engaging, interactive process. You'll see how prayer affects the mind of the prayer.

We also need to pray when we're grateful. Gratefulness means great fullness in our hearts. My granddaughter Grace had a diving accident and I accompanied her in the ambulance as she was rushed to the hospital. As she was strapped down on the gurney, I began praying out loud for her and the anxious EMTs. Thankfully, Grace regained all sensation in her legs and didn't suffer a permanent injury. The next day, Larry and I demonstrated for Elijah and Grace how to celebrate and praise God for our blessings. This was a simple way to leave our values and mentor the next generation of loved ones.

We are meant to continually evolve in conscious awareness and to grow spiritually as we age. As our pace slows, we have more time and interest to explore the inner landscape of our souls. The demands of work and social obligations decrease. In their place, we relax into becoming more accepting of all circumstances. We become more keenly aware of focusing on and being thankful for all that we have. We're definitely more aware of the finiteness of life. In quiet moments, we tend to our growing souls as we see chances to blossom into our fully unique ripe beauty. We discover the gifts of our authentic self.

## Facing Death and Finding Life

"It is impossible that anything so natural, so necessary, and so universal as death, should ever have been designed by providence as an evil to mankind."

—JONATHAN SWIFT

In a unique twist of fate, when I was diagnosed with hep C and doomed to die, I really never felt more aware of and grateful for my life—and all life, for that matter. Even though I felt awful in my body, and was suffering from unbelievable fatigue and discomfort.

The reality of death gets us up real close to the flip side of how precious life is. Early on in the Judds' Farewell Tour, a woman with breast cancer came onto the bus and shared that her cancer was the best thing that ever happened to her. Wy wondered out loud if her disease had affected her brain! But having been through the dark night of the soul myself, I get it. When we acknowledge that there are simply no guarantees for any of us, and that it could suddenly be over, we get clear about our priorities. We start seeing lots of chances to live life in the moment. It's liberating and expansive!

At age thirty, Steve Jobs, the inventor of the Macintosh computer and founder of Apple, got fired from his own company in a very public and messy takeover. Embarrassed and devastated for a while, he slunk into a well of misery and self-pity. But Steve was flexible enough to start over. His elevated consciousness tipped him off: "The heaviness of being successful can be replaced by the lightness of being a beginner again." He bravely entered into the most creative state of his life, starting NeXT and Pixar, the creators of *Toy Story* and other hugely successful films.

Then Steve was diagnosed with pancreatic cancer and given three months to live. Suddenly he saw that embarrassment and fear of failure—all these powerful self-defeating emotions—fell away in the face of impending death. He confesses, "Remembering that you will die is the best way to avoid the rap of thinking you have something to lose." It dawned on him in a dramatic way how limited time actually is and was glad he hadn't ever wasted a drop trying to live someone else's life. Steve had been following his heart all along. However, he suddenly had only a couple of months to tell his wife and kids everything he assumed he'd have another decade or two to express. In a stunning reversal of fortune, a biopsy revealed that he had a very rare, curable form of pancreatic cancer. Now cured by surgery, Steve tells everyone that death is "the single best invention of life. It's Life's Change Agent." I don't want you to have to go through what Steve and I have in order to realize you can live by your heart every minute of every day. Don't ever give energy to thinking about what could go wrong or what you could lose.

When we choose to face our inevitable mortality, we plug the energy drain that's caused by denying it. Free yourself up right now to go full steam in facing reality. Begin doing something wonderful, useful, with however much time you have left!

Hold a quarter tightly in your fist with your palm facing down. It takes energy to keep it from dropping, right? Now turn your palm over and open your hand. The coin stays there with virtually no effort on your part. When you're denying your mortality, you're spending energy holding yourself together. When we just admit it, thoughts become easier. Accepting death is like an open hand rather than a tight fist.

Researchers studying those who live to a hundred and beyond find that they choose to deal sensibly with any feelings that come up around their mortality. It's not that they don't have fears. But they learn to relax and cope with their fears instead of dwelling on them. They remember that there have been other crises in their lives that came and went. They find ways to continue to be flexible, enjoy simple little things, and contribute to others.

Death is our last great mystery. How about allowing yourself to have curiosity and anticipation? It's even okay that no one knows exactly what will happen. No one.

My friend Carl Perkins, the great rockabilly musician and creator of "Blue Suede Shoes," called me right before he died. "Honey," he admitted, "it's like when you got hepatitis C. I was so angry at God and I thought, boy, I can't wait to get to heaven and ask why do we suffer. Then it dawned on me once I see the face of God, these questions won't even be relevant." Carl reminded me that the Bible says we'll recognize each other in heaven.

You can also get insights from the reports of near-death experiences describing peaceful sensations of seeing light and of meeting all whom you loved that have gone before you. A thought-provoking book on the topic is *Life After Life* by Raymond Moody, a physician who surveyed hundreds of near-death experiences. The people experienced an overwhelming sense of unconditional love. Think of it this way—this human experience is only a stage of our eternal existence, with death the transition to the next stage. Consider these beautiful lines from John Keats: "A thing of beauty is a joy for ever; its loveliness increases; it will never pass into nothingness." After four decades of work in the field of death and dying, Elisabeth Kübler-Ross, who passed away in 2004, began studying near-death experiences. "When we leave the physical body," she wrote, "we experience a physical wholeness in the 'ethereal body.' This temporary body that we have when we experience the scene of our own death has no pain and no handicaps. If we have been amputees, we will have our limbs again; if we have been deaf, we can hear."

Elisabeth Kübler-Ross, Thich Nhat Hanh, Ram Dass, and many other world mentors of compassion speak about the transition in *Graceful Passages: A Companion for Living & Dying,* a spoken-word CD with heart-opening music packaged with a gift book. Through music and a series of readings drawing on a variety of religious traditions, it takes the listener on a gentle journey of the higher perspective of death and dying. I recommend it for terminally ill individuals and their families, especially folks who are unsure how to begin a dialogue. I'm a supporter of hospice and I hear from members of this fine organization that most distraught families have no idea how to discuss what's happening.

## Where There's a Will, There's a Way

"Our freedom comes in the way we accept things over which we have no control . . . even death."
—MADELEINE L'ENGLE

One way we can help ourselves and our family members not fear death is to anticipate and get ready for it just like we plan for any major milestone. Have you written your will and signed the organ donor card? How about filling out the papers for durable power of attorney and medical durable power of attorney so that if you can't make your own decisions, your wishes will be respected? I sure have! My sister Margaret and I took that burden off our husbands and children by each agreeing to be the one to enforce the other's wishes.

What I saw as an RN in the ICU led me to decide against heroic measures to bring patients back after their hearts stop in end-of-life situations. I'm a believer in DNR (do not resuscitate) orders when the end is near. Eighty percent of health-care costs are incurred in the last two months of life. Reread that statistic and tell it to someone else! Life is made up of choices and this is your last one. Make yours known this week, before that choice is taken away from you!

Well, here's another cheery consideration: Have you given thought to what you'd like your funeral to be? I want mine to be a celebration! I've designated the six pallbearers and one alternate, and put together a list of my favorite music. Since the Judds have and always will be about audience participation, I invite people to share with my family stories about any encounters or connection they had with me.

The average funeral costs $6,000. It's a well-organized industry with its own lobbyists. These businessmen and -women can be clever in playing on people's vulnerability in their worst crisis. That's why I urge you to consider your choices well in advance. Do it today.

Living in the country, we appreciate natural processes. At the funeral of our neighbor Harding Meachum, Larry, Wy, Roach, and I went to the rural cemetery, where some of Harding's fellow farmers dug his grave. Birds and butterflies landed on the casket as a breeze stirred. It reminded me of services for my Judd grandparents, aunts, and uncles. As they lowered him down into the earth Harding lived so close to all his days, I smiled, because that's just the way it's supposed to be.

# When the Night Is Darkest, That's When the Stars Come Out

"When you're fifty, you start thinking about things you haven't thought about before. I used to think getting old was about vanity—but actually it's about losing people you love. Getting wrinkles is trivial."

—JOYCE CAROL OATES

The longer we live, the more we will go through the loss of loved ones. That's just one of the facts of life.

The predictable stages of grief are denial, anger, guilt, depression, acceptance, and growth. It's very beneficial to understand these stages to steer us through the fog of confusion. You may feel several of these emotions at once because it's not necessarily a process from one stage to the other. How long each step goes on varies from person to person. One fact to take comfort in is that it does get better over time.

Studies of those who live to a hundred show that they have developed an amazing ability to deal with the stress of grief. They don't deny their grief or sadness; they accept death as another part of life. Many rely on their faith to give comfort that their beloved is in another realm. They also seek to find meaning in the loss.

It's also about what we choose to do with our feelings about death. My brother Mark became a pastor in the wake of our brother Brian's death. Brian's best friend, Jimmy Lett, was so affected by Brian's early passing that he became a doctor. I felt really helpless, and I believe that is why I became a nurse.

The following eight tips from the National Hospice and Palliative Care Organization offer help for dealing with grief.

1    **Feel the Pain**

Give into it—even give it precedence over other emotions and activities, because grief is a pain that will get in your way later if it is ignored. Grief has no timetable; it is cyclical, so expect emotions to come and go for weeks, months, or even years. While a show of strength is admirable, it does not serve the powerful need to express sadness, even when it comes out at unexpected times and places.

2    **Talk About Your Sorrow**

Take the time to seek comfort from friends who will listen. Let them know you need to talk about your loss. People will understand, although they may not know how to respond. If they change the subject, bring them back to your need to share your memories and express your sorrow.

3    **Forgive Yourself**

Forgive yourself for all you believe you should have said or done. Also forgive yourself for any anger, guilt, and embarrassment you feel while grieving.

4    **Eat Well and Exercise**

Grief is exhausting. To sustain energy, maintain a balanced diet by regular meals. Exercise is also important in sustaining energy. Find a routine that suits you—perhaps walks or bike rides with friends, or in solitude. Moving your body clears your mind and refreshes your body.

5    **Indulge Yourself**

Take naps, read a good book, get out in nature, listen to your favorite music, get a massage, go to a ball game, attend church, rent a movie, volunteer at your favorite charity. Do something that is frivolous, distracting, and comforting.

**6    Prepare for Holidays and Anniversaries**

Expect to feel especially blue during periods like the anniversary date of the death. Even if you think you've progressed, these dates may bring back painful emotions. Make arrangements to be with friends and family members with whom you are at ease. Plan some type of ceremony to release your emotions.

**7    Get Help**

Bereavement groups can help you recognize your feelings and then put them in perspective. They can also help alleviate feeling you are alone. The experience of sharing with others in a similar situation can be quite comforting and reassuring. Sometimes, new friendships grow through these groups—even a whole new social network. Check with your local hospice or other bereavement support groups for more information. If you find that you are in great distress or in long-term depression, individual or group therapy from a counselor who specializes in grief may be advisable.

**8    Take Active Steps to Create a New Phase**

Give yourself as much time to grieve as you need. Once you find some new energy, begin to look for one interesting thing to do. Take a course, donate time to a cause you support, meet new people.

In dealing with losses of all kinds, I have come to understand not to take loss personally. Losses happen to everyone. They offer us the choice to expand instead of contract, and to get an idea of what's going on with others. Grief ultimately offers us the choice we would not have had to grow our souls. It's a time to connect intimately with God, to find new strength, to connect to whatever deeply matters to us.

Crisis helps us reach new conclusions and experiment. I would not have gone on the journey of investigating the mind/body/spirit connection if I hadn't suffered through the prognosis of a terminal illness. And I would not have developed my inner resources. I came upon greater resilience and ultimately peace of mind. The increased awareness we are forced into by grief is one of our greatest legacies as human beings. It not only makes us stronger, but the wisdom, empathy, and compassion we gain are invaluable gifts we have to pass on to others. Peace of mind is the ultimate goal.

## Your Turn Now

- If you're a believer, are you keeping your God connection strong? Do you say grace at meals? Go to church? Pray daily? Communicate with others who believe as you do? Do you use your faith to help you through hard times? How about starting every morning in solitude, getting centered in your beliefs?

- What are your feelings about your death? What is your greatest fear? Is there something practical you can do to alleviate it? Do you believe the soul lives on?

- Describe the funeral or memorial service that you would like for yourself. Do you want to be buried or cremated? What kind of music do you want? Whom do you want to speak? What prayers, poems, and other readings would you like? Who should be there? Where should it take place? Whom do you want to be pallbearers? Make sure your loved ones know your wishes.

- Have you signed documents to protect yourself medically and financially if you become incapable of taking care of yourself? There are two forms: durable power of attorney (which gives someone else control over your money) and medical power of attorney (often referred to as a living will). These forms vary from state to state. Be sure that you clearly understand what you are signing up for. You may want to consult an attorney. To get a free medical power of attorney form, also called advance directive, for your state, go to www.caringinfo.org. It offers a wide range of materials that relate to end-of-life care, caregiving, grief, and advance care planning.

- If you or someone you love is dying (or going through another painful transition), you might like to order *Graceful Passages*. It is available at www.wisdomoftheworld.com or www.amazon.com.

- Fill out an organ donor card and tell someone you know to do it also. Eight people die every day waiting for a liver. You can literally give the gift of life to someone.

- To find a hospice program near you, go to www.hospice.net or call the National Hospice Organization at 800-646-6460.

- Create an ethical will to pass on your values. This is a nonlegal document in which you express your beliefs, the most important things life has taught you, and your wishes for your loved ones. It can be as short as a paragraph or as long as a book. When I wrote my autobiography, *Love Can Build a Bridge,* I dedicated it "to my future Grandchildren and their descendants. This is who we are and how we lived."

- Your ethical will can be videotaped or put down on acid-free paper and placed in a special scrapbook to be preserved for generations to come. One way to do it is to have a young relative—a grandchild, a niece—to interview you about your life on video- or audiotape. Transcribe the tapes and voilà! Find out more by reading *Ethical Wills* by Barry Baines, MD. If you want more support, visit www.personalhistorians.org, which will help you find a professional to assist in creating your own unique ethical will.

- How do you want to help younger folks? One place to begin is to ask yourself the question that Rabbi Schachter-Shalomi suggests: "What would I grieve for if I failed to transmit it?" After you've got your list, ask yourself, "Who are the likely people to benefit from my experiences?" Then go find them.

"Make wisdom your provision for the journey from youth to old age, for it is a more certain support than all other possessions."
—BIAS

# 11 | Parting Wishes

NOW, YOU'VE READ MY MIND. It's my deepest wish that, by sharing some of my own experiences of aging, I'm passing on something of value to take with you into this most meaningful phase of your life. So get psyched about exploring our new frontier of healthy, happy longevity. Researchers predict that our generation will live longer on average than any other in history. We don't get to choose when we are born or when we will die. Our tombstones will proclaim the dates of our birth and death. It's totally up to us how we choose to live the part in between. Live every day as if it's your last, 'cause one day it will be.

Carl Jung said "You are a soul. You have a body." The older I get, the more aware of this I become. This is one of the best benefits of aging. Self-awareness shows us how we can see everything in our lives as a chance to grow our souls. When we embrace this perspective, our way of thinking becomes deeper, richer, and more satisfying. That's why I know that everything is actually a spiritual problem with a spiritual solution. Armed with that truth, along with open-minded, positive attitudes about a new style of aging, lighter loads, a stronger sense of purpose, a support network of friends and family, a deep connection to God, and lots of laughter and moisturizer, we should be just fine.

You're the author of the story of your life. Every day your choices are making up the plots and you are choosing the cast of characters. The end of the last chapter is just the beginning of your soul's never-ending story.

Signed,
The New Older Woman

# ACKNOWLEDGMENTS

Awareness of what we have to be grateful for is the foundation for remaining content throughout the many phases and stages of life. That's why I chose to use the term "aging gratefully," in the title of this book as opposed to the more common "aging gracefully."

So I would like to acknowledge my gratitude to Amanda Murray at Simon & Schuster for encouraging me to write this book. And Nancy Inglis, Kristan Fletcher, Annie Orr, Cynthia Merman, Donna Rivera, Philip Bashe, and the staff at Simon & Schuster for their hard work.

Also, to the godfather of literary agents and a good friend who makes me laugh, Mel Berger at the William Morris Agency.

To Mary Jane Ryan, who did the meticulous research and helped keep me focused (no easy task). This book wouldn't have happened without you.

And finally to Alma Wiggins, an African-American senior citizen working as the attendant in the ladies' room at the Wilshire Regency Hotel in Beverly Hills. Chatting with her about getting older, I mentioned that I was writing a book pointing out the good aspects of aging and reporting new data on living longer and healthier. She looked at me square in the eye and pleaded: "Tell folks that I may be older but I'm still a human being with feelings. They shouldn't act like I'm invisible when they pass me on the street."

# SELECTED BIBLIOGRAPHY

Achat, H., I. Kawachi, S. Levine, C. Berkey, E. Coakley, and G. Colditz. 1998. "Social Networks, Stress and Health-Related Quality of Life." *Quality of Life Research* 7:735–50.

Anderson, Norman B. *Emotional Longevity.* New York: Viking, 2003.

Arora, Raksha, and Lydia Saad. "Marketing to Older Affluents." *Gallup Management Journal,* June 9, 2005.

Baran, Josh. *365 Nirvana.* London: Element, 2003.

Baron, John A., et al. 2003. "A Randomized Trial of Aspirin to Prevent Colorectal Adenomas." *The New England Journal of Medicine* 348:891–99.

Bauer, Joy. "Boost Your Metabolism and Lose Weight Faster." MSNBC "Today's Health," July 18, 2006.

Beers, Mark H., ed. *The Merck Manual of Health & Aging.* Whitehouse Station, NJ: Merck Research Laboratories, 2004.

Bennett, Gary G., Kathleen Y. Wolin, K. Viswanath, Sandy Askew, Elaine Puleo, and Karen M. Emmons, "Television Viewing and Pedometer-Determined Physical Activity Among Multiethnic Residents of Low-Income Housing." *American Journal of Public Health* 96:1681–85.

Bielby, Denise and Bill. "Hollywood Ageism Persists." *Back to 93106* 13, no. 10 (February 2003).

Boothby, L.A., and P.L. Doering. "Vitamin C and Vitamin E for Alzheimer's Disease." *Annals of Pharmacotherapy* 39:2073–80.

Bortz, Walter M., II. *Dare to Be 100.* New York: Fireside, 1996.

Boyd, Clem, and Roberta Rand. "Ageism in Hollywood." *Focus Over Fifty,* 2002. www.family.org.focusoverfifty/articles/a0021893.cfm.

Brehony, Kathleen A. *Awakening at Midlife.* New York: Riverhead Books, 1996.

Brody, Jane. "Aging and Infirmity: Twinned No Longer." *New York Times,* January 25, 2005.

Brown, Brene. *Women & Shame: Reaching Out, Speaking Truths and Building Connections.* Austin, TX: 3C Press, 2004.

Carter, Jimmy. *The Virtues of Aging.* New York: Ballantine, 1998.

Centerwall, B. "Television and Violence: The Scale of the Problem and Where to Go from Here." *Journal of the American Medical Association* 267:3059–61.

Cilley, Marla. *Sink Reflections.* New York: Bantam Books, 2002.

Cisek, Edward, and Kathleen Triche. "Depression and Social Support Among Older Adult Computer Users." Presentation made at 113th Annual Convention of the American Psychological Association, Washington, DC, August 18, 2005.

Cohen, Elizabeth. "Your Parents Are Getting Older. Are You Ready?" *Redbook,* February 2005.

Cohen, Gene D. "The Creativity and Aging Study: The Impact of Professionally Conducted Cultural Programs on Older Adults." Final Report: April 2006.

Comfort, Alex. *A Good Age.* New York: Crown Publishers, 1976.

Committee on Assuring the Health of the Public in the 21st Century.
*The Future of the Public's Health in the 21st Century.* Washington, DC:
The National Academies Press, 2002.

Coombes, Andrea. "Aging Boomers Fight for Entertainment Limelight."
*CBS MarketWatch,* March 4, 2004.

Corrada, Maria M., Claudia H. Kawas, Judith Hallfrisch, Denis Muller, and
Ron Brookmeyer. "Reduced Risk of Alzheimer's Disease with High
Folate Intake: The Baltimore Longitudinal Study of Aging." *Alzheimer's
& Dementia* 1:11–18.

"Could an Aspirin a Day Help Keep Prostate Cancer Away? Possibly."
*Science Daily,* March 13, 2002. (online)

Cowell, J.A. "Aspirin for the Primary Prevention of Cardiovascular Events."
*Drugs Today* 42:467–79.

Crowley, Chris, and Henry S. Lodge. *Younger Next Year.* New York:
Workman, 2005.

Davis, Susan R., Sonia L. Davison, Susan Donath, and Robin J. Bell.
"Circulating Androgen Levels and Self-Reported Sexual Function
in Women." *Journal of the American Medical Association* 294:91–96.

"Deaths: Leading Causes for Mortality 2003." *National Vital Statistics Report,*
National Center for Health Statistics.

Delehanty, Hugh. "The Care Dividend." *AARP Magazine,* May and June
2005.

Department of Health and Human Services (HHS) and the Department of
Agriculture (USDA). *Dietary Guidelines for Americans 2005.*

Derenne, Jennifer L., and Eugene V. Beresin. "Body Image, Media, and
Eating Disorders." *Academic Psychiatry* 30:257–61.

Donlon, Margie M., Ori Ashman, and Becca R. Levy. "Re-vision of Older Television Characters: A Stereotype-Awareness Intervention." *Journal of Social Issues* 61:307.

Dowling, John E. *The Great Brain Debate.* Washington, DC: John Henry Press, 2004.

Dychtwald, Ken. *Age Power.* New York: Jeremy P. Tarcher/Putnam, 1999.

Dye, Lee. "Study: Exercise and Music Clear the Brain." ABC News Online, April 1, 2006.

Easterbrook, Gregg. "Rx for Life: Gratitude." www.beliefnet.com/story/51/story_5111_html.

Emmons, Robert. "Highlights from the Research Project on Gratitude and Thankfulness." http://psychology.ucdavis.edu/labs/emmons/.

Emmons, Robert A., and Michael E. McCullough. "Counting Blessings versus Burdens: Experimental Studies of Gratitude and Subjective Well-Being in Daily Life. *Journal of Personality and Social Psychology* 84:377–389.

Epel, E.S., B. McEwen, T. Seeman, K. Matthews, G. Castellazzo, K.D. Brownell, J. Bell, and J.R. Ickovics. "Stress and Body Shape: Stress-Induced Cortisol Secretion Is Consistently Greater Among Women with Central Fat." *Psychosomatic Medicine* 62:623–32.

Escobar-Chaves, S. Liliana. "Impact of the Media on Adolescent Sexual Attitudes and Behaviors." *Pediatrics* 116:ii.

Farshchi, Hamid R., Moria A. Taylor, and Ian A. Macdonald. "Deleterious Effects of Omitting Breakfast on Insulin Sensitivity and Fasting Lipid Profiles in Healthy Lean Women." *American Journal of Clinical Nutrition* 81(2):388–96.

"Female Fertility Drug May Combat Age-Related Male Testosterone Deficiency: Columbia Presbyterian Researchers Evaluate New

Therapy," Columbia University Health Sciences press release, May 2003.

Fisch, Harry. *The Male Biological Clock.* New York: Free Press, 2005.

Frank, B., and S. Gupta. "A Review of Antioxidants and Alzheimer's Disease." *Annals of Clinical Psychiatry* 17:269–86.

Gentile, Gary. "Fighting Ageism in Hollywood." www.cbsnews.com/stories/2002/08/01/entertainment/main517206.shtml.

Gertz, Kathryn Rose. "Why Laughter Is Good for You." *Family Circle*, January 18, 2005.

Giltay, Erik J., Johanna M. Geleijnse, Frans G. Zitman, Tiny Hoekstra, and Evert G. Schouten. "Dispositional Optimism and All-cause and Cardiovascular Mortality in a Prospective Cohort of Elderly Dutch Men and Women." *Archives of General Psychiatry* 61:1126–35.

Giltay, E.J., M.H. Kamphuis, S. Kalmijn, F.G. Zitman, and D. Kromhout. "Dispositional Optimism and the Risk of Cardiovascular Death: The Zutphen Elderly Study." *Archives of Internal Medicine* 166:431–36.

Giovannucci, E., and M. Pollak. "Risk of Cancer after Growth-Hormone Treatment." *The Lancet* 360:268–69.

Goldbeck, Nikki and David. *The Good Breakfast Book.* Woodstock, NY: Ceres Press, 1992.

Goleman, Daniel. "Finding Happiness: Cajole Your Brain to Lean to the Left." *New York Times,* February 4, 2003.

Gonzalez, Alejandro J., Emily White, Alan Kristal, and Alyson J. Littman. "Calcium Intake and 10-Year Weight Change in Middle-aged Adults." *Journal of the American Dietetic Association* 106:1066–1073.

"Grandparenting." www.helpguide.org/mental/grandparenting.htm.

Greene, Roberta R., and Jirina S. Polivka. "The Meaning of Grandparents' Day Cards: An Analysis of the Intergenerational Network." *Family Relations* 34:221–25.

Hales, Dianne. "Why Prayer Could Be Good Medicine." *Parade* magazine, March 23, 2003.

Hall, Daniel E. "Religious Attendance: More Cost-Effective Than Lipitor?" *Journal of the American Board of Family Medicine* 19:103–109.

Hancock, Elise. "A Primer on Touch." *Johns Hopkins Magazine,* electronic edition, September 1996.

Hargrave, Terry. "When You're 64: A New Model for Caregiving." *Psychotherapy Networker,* July/August 2005.

Hess, John L. "Geezer-Bashing: Media Attacks on the Elderly." *Fairness & Accuracy In Reporting,* July/August 1991. www.fair.org/index.php?page-1511.

Holmes, Bob, et al. "Reasons to Be Cheerful." *New Scientist,* October 4, 2003.

International Longevity Center-USA, Ltd. "Longevity Genes: Hunting for the Secrets of the Super Centenarians." AARP Foundation, 2004.

——. "Older People Hardier, More Productive Than Stereotypes Suggest." *Age Boom Observer,* November 9, 2000.

Janal, Dan. "Ageism and the Media." E-newsletter, February 16, 2005.

Johnson, Paula A. "Health Disparities in Cardiovascular Disease."

Johnson, Richard P. *The 12 Keys to Spiritual Vitality.* Liguori, MO: Liguori, 1998.

Kaiser Family Foundation. *The Media Family,* November 2005. www.kff.org/entmedia/7500/cfm.

Kanigel, Rachele. "Too Much Information!" *Organic Style,* November 2004.

Klatz, Ronald, and Robert Goldman. *The New Anti-Aging Revolution.* North Bergen, NJ: Basic Health Publications, 2003.

Kornhaber, Arthur. "That Vital Connection: Grandparents as Spiritual Guides." Foundation for Grandparenting. www.grandparenting.org.

Kubzansky, L.D., D. Sparrow, P. Vokonas, and I. Kawachi. "Is the Glass Half Empty or Half Full? A Prospective Study of Optimism and Coronary Heart Disease in the Normative Aging Study." *Psychosomatic Medicine* 63:910–16.

Lambert, Craig. "Deep into Sleep." *Harvard Magazine,* July–August 2005.

Lee, David. "Whatever Life Brings." www.HumanNatureatWork.com.

Leider, Richard J., and David A. Shapiro. *Claiming Your Place at the Fire.* San Francisco: Berrett-Koehler, 2004.

Lemonick, Michael D. "The Biology of Joy." *Time,* January 17, 2005.

———. "The Ravages of Stress." *Time,* December 13, 2004.

Lennartsson, Carin. "Social Ties and Health Among the Very Old in Sweden." *Research on Aging* 21:657–81.

Levine, Suzanne Braun. *Inventing the Rest of Our Lives.* New York: Viking, 2005.

Levy, B. "Improving Memory in Old Age Through Implicit Self-stereotyping." *Journal of Personality and Social Psychology* 71:1092–1107.

Levy, B.R., J. Hausdorff, R. Hencke, and J. Wei. "Reducing Cardiovascular Stress with Positive Self-Stereotypes of Aging." *The Journals of Gerontology Series B: Psychological Sciences and Social Science* 55:205–13.

Levy, B.R., M.D. Slade, S.R. Kunkel, and S.V. Kasl. "Longevity Increased by Positive Self-Perceptions of Aging." *Journal of Personality and Social Psychology* 83:261–70.

Little, Jeni. "Whole-Person Health Care." *Duke Magazine*, September–
October 2002.

Mahoney, David, and Richard Restak. *The Longevity Strategy*. New York: John
Wiley, 1998.

Martinez, Iveris L., Kevin Frick, Thomas A. Glass, Michelle Carlson,
Elizabeth Tanner, Michelle Ricks, and Linda P. Fried. "Engaging
Older Adults in High Impact Volunteering That Enhances Health:
Recruitment and Retention in the Experience Corps, Baltimore."
*Journal of Urban Health* 83(4):online.

Matthews, Dale. *The Faith Factor*. New York: Viking, 1998.

McKhann, Guy, and Marilyn Albert. *Keep Your Brain Young*. New York: John
Wiley, 2003.

Molla, Michael T., Diane K. Wagener, and Jennifer H. Madans. "Summary
Measures of Population Health: Methods for Calculating Healthy Life
Expectancy." Centers for Disease Control and Prevention. *Healthy
People 2010, Statistical Notes*, number 21.

Moran, Victoria. *Younger by the Day*. San Francisco: Harper, 2004.

Morris, M.C., D.A. Evans, C.C. Tangey, J.L. Bienias, and R.S. Wilson. "Fish
Consumption and Cognitive Decline with Age in a Large Community
Study." *Archives of Neurology* 62:1849–53.

National Sleep Foundation. "How to Get a Good Night's Sleep."
www.sleepfoundation.org.

"National Vital Statistics Report. Deaths: Leading Causes for Mortality 2003.
Preliminary Data for 2003." National Center for Health Statistics,
2006.

Newton, Diana Carney. "Staying Close to Grandkids Who Live Far Away."
San Diego, CA: Eldercare Directory. http://eldercare.uniontrib.com/
news/news/-grands.cfm.

Norat, Teresa, et al. "Meat, Fish, and Colorectal Cancer Risk: The European Prospective Investigation into Cancer and Nutrition." *Journal of the National Cancer Institute* 97:906–16.

Northcott, H.T.C. "Too Young, too Old: Age in the World of Television." *The Gerontologist* 15:184–86.

Northrup, Christiane. *Mother-Daughter Wisdom.* New York: Bantam Books, 2005.

Okinawa Centenarian Study. http://okinawaprogram.com/study.html.

"Oldest Baby Boomers Turn 60!" U.S. Census Bureau, January 3, 2006. http://www.census.gov/Press-Release/www/releases/archives/facts_for_features_special_editions/006105.html.

Pantuck, Allan J., et al. "Phase II Study of Pomegranate Juice for Men with Rising Prostate-Specific Antigen Following Surgery or Radiation for Prostate Cancer." *Clinical Cancer Research* 12:4018–26.

Parents Television Council. E-Alert, vol. 3, no. 18.

Park, Andrew. "Between a Rocker and a High Chair." *BusinessWeek,* February 21, 2005.

Peeke, Pamela. *Body-for-LIFE for Women.* Emmaus, PA: Rodale, 2005.

———. *Fight Fat After Forty.* New York: Penguin Books, 2000.

Peeke, P.M., and G.P. Chrousos. "Hypercortisolism and Obesity." *Annals of the New York Academy of Sciences* 771:665–76.

Perls, Thomas T. "Who Are Centenarians?" http://www.med.harvard.edu/programs/necs/centenarians.htm.

Perls, Thomas T., and Margery Hutter Silver. *Living to 100.* New York: Basic Books, 1999.

Petty, David L. *Aging Gracefully.* Nashville: Broadman & Holman, 2003.

Pipher, Mary. *Another Country.* New York: Riverhead Books, 1999.

Pittman, Frank. "Beware: Older Women Ahead." *Psychology Today,* January 1999.

Piver, Susan. *The Hard Questions for Adult Children and Their Aging Parents.* New York: Gotham, 2004.

Popov, Linda Kavelin. *A Pace for Grace.* New York: Plume, 2004.

Potempa, Ann. "Get Wed, Live Longer." *Anchorage Daily News,* February 15, 2006.

Prior, Molly. "Dove Ad Campaign Aims to Redefine Beauty." *Women's Wear Daily,* October 8, 2004.

Ram Dass. *Still Here.* New York: Riverhead Books, 2000.

Ramirez, Eddy. "Ageism in the Media Is Seen as Harmful to Health of Elderly." *Los Angeles Times,* September 5, 2002.

"Red Meat Doubles Rheumatoid Arthritis Risk." Medical News Today (online), December 6, 2004.

Reynolds, Gretchen. "PHYS ED; Raging Hormones." *The New York Times,* August 20, 2006.

Ritchie, Ed. "Forgiveness Can Be Healthy." National Fibromyalgia Association. www.fmaware.org/patient/coping/forgiveness/htm.

Robinson, Barrie. "Ageism." University of California, Berkeley, School of Social Welfare, 1994.

Roizen, Michael F., and Mehmet C. Oz. *You: The Owner's Manual.* New York: HarperCollins, 2005.

Rosenblatt, Roger. *Rules for Aging.* San Diego: Harcourt, 2000.

Ryan, M. J. *Attitudes of Gratitude.* Berkeley, CA: Conari Press, 1999.

——. *The Giving Heart.* Berkeley, CA: Conari Press, 2000.

——. *The Happiness Makeover.* New York: Broadway Books, 2005.

Schachter-Shalomi, Zalman. *From Age-ing to Sage-ing.* New York: Warner, 1995.

Schernhammer, E.S., J.H. Kang, A.T. Chan, D.S. Michaud, H.G. Skinner, E. Giovannucci, G.A. Colditz, and C.S. Fuchs. "A Prospective Study of Aspirin Use and the Risk of Pancreatic Cancer in Women." *Journal of the National Cancer Institute* 96:22–28.

Schulz, Mona Lisa. *The New Feminine Brain: Developing Your Intuitive Genius.* New York: Free Press, 2003.

Schwartz, Lisa M., Steven Woloshin, and H. Gilbert Welch. "Overstating Aspirin's Role in Breast Cancer Prevention." *Washington Post,* May 10, 2005.

Shults, Clifford W., et al. "Effects of Coenzyme Q10 in Early Parkinson Disease: Evidence of Slowing of the Functional Decline." *Archives of Neurology* 59:1541–50.

The Science of Happiness Special Mind & Body Issue. *Time,* January 17, 2005.

Scott-Clark, Cathy, and Adrian Levy. "Fast Forward into Trouble." *The Guardian,* June 14, 2003.

See, Carolyn. "Gift of a Lifetime." *AARP The Magazine,* September–October 2004.

Seligman, Martin. *Authentic Happiness.* New York: Free Press, 2002.

——. *Learned Optimism.* New York: Vintage, 1999.

"Sexuality at Midlife and Beyond: 2004 Update of Attitudes and Behaviors." Commissioned by *AARP,* 2005.

"Size Matters: Shortest Telomeres Initiate Cellular Havoc." JHMI Office of Communications and Public Affairs, October 5, 2001. (press release)

Small, Gary W., et al. "Effects of a 14-Day Healthy Longevity Lifestyle Program on Cognition and Brain Function." *American Journal of Geriatric Psychiatry* 14:538–45.

Snowdon, David. *Aging with Grace.* New York: Bantam, 2001.

John Sparks. "The Singing-Health Connection." Chorus America. www .chorusamerica.org/vox_article_singinghealth.cfm.

Starr, Bernard. "It Ain't Just the Paint: Aging and the Media." Speech to the American Society on Aging, March 1997.

Swanbrow, Diane. "Forgiveness May Lead to Better Health." *The University Record On-line,* December 17, 2001. http://www.umich.edu/~urecord/ archives.shtml.

Taylor, S.E., L.C. Klein, B.P. Lewis, T.L. Gruenewald, R.A. Gurung, and J.A. Updegraff. "Female Responses to Stress: Tend and Befriend, Not Fight or Flight." *Psychological Review* 107:411–29.

"Teens and Their Parents in the 21st Century: An Examination of Trends in Teen Behavior and the Role of Parental Involvement." The Council of Economic Advisors, 2000.

Tolson, Chester L., and Harold George Koenig. *The Healing Power of Prayer.* Grand Rapids, MI: Baker Books, 2003.

Toussaint, L.L, D.R. Williams, M.A. Musick, and S.A. Everson. "Forgiveness and Health: Age Differences in a U.S. Probability Sample." *Journal of Adult Development* 8:249–57.

Tsai, Shan P., Judy K. Wendt, Robin P. Donnelly, Geert de Jong, and Farah S. Ahmed. "Age at Retirement and Long-term Survival of an Industrial Population: Prospective Cohort Study." *British Medical Journal* 331:995.

Tupper, Meredith. "The Representation of Elderly Persons in Primetime Television Advertising." Master's thesis, University of South Florida, School of Mass Communications, November 1995.

Vaillant, George. *Aging Well.* Boston: Little, Brown, 2002.

Ward, Sela. *Oprah,* March 17, 2000.

Weil, Andrew. *Healthy Aging.* New York: Knopf, 2005.

Westberg, Granger. *Good Grief.* Minneapolis: Augsberg Fortress, 1997.

White, Ken. "Senior Actors Call on Hollywood to End Ageism." *Las Vegas Review-Journal,* June 15, 2000.

Willcox, Bradley J., D. Craig Willcox, and Makoto Suzuki. *The Okinawa Program.* New York: Three Rivers Press, 2002.

Williams, Kristi. "Has the Future of Marriage Arrived? A Contemporary Examination of Gender, Marriage, and Psychological Well-being." *Journal of Health and Social Behavior* 44:470–87.

Williams, Kristi, and Debra Umberson. "Marital Status, Marital Transitions and Health: A Gendered Life Course Perspective." *Journal of Health and Social Behavior* 45:81–98.

Willis, Clint. "Have 'The Talk' with Your Parents." *Money,* April 1, 2005.

Woolf, Linda. "Ageism Empirical Evidence." www.webster.edu/~woolflm/ageismempirical.html.

Wright, Robert. "Dancing to Evolution's Tune." *Time,* January 17, 2005.

# INDEX